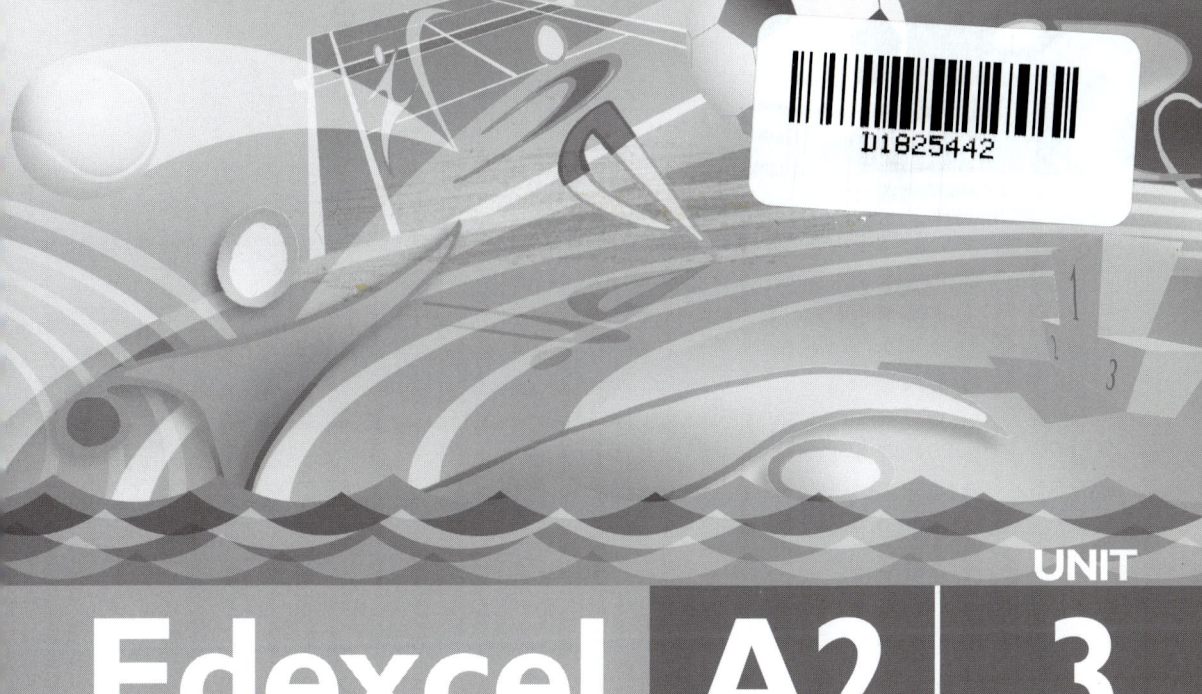

UNIT

Edexcel A2 | 3

Physical Education

Preparation for Optimum Sports Performance

Mike Hill and Gavin Roberts

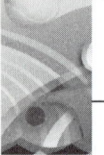
Philip Allan Updates, an imprint of Hodder Education, an Hachette UK company, Market Place, Deddington, Oxfordshire OX15 0SE

Orders

Bookpoint Ltd, 130 Milton Park, Abingdon, Oxfordshire OX14 4SB
tel: 01235 827720
fax: 01235 400454
e-mail: uk.orders@bookpoint.co.uk
Lines are open 9.00 a.m.–5.00 p.m., Monday to Saturday, with a 24-hour message answering service. You can also order through the Philip Allan Updates website: www.philipallan.co.uk

© Philip Allan Updates 2009

ISBN 978-0-340-96678-5

First printed 2009
Impression number 5 4 3 2 1
Year 2014 2013 2012 2011 2010 2009

This guide has been written specifically to support students preparing for the Edexcel A2 Physical Education Unit 3 examination. The content has been neither approved nor endorsed by Edexcel and remains the sole responsibility of the authors.

Typeset by Phoenix Photosetting, Chatham, Kent
Printed by MPG Books, Bodmin

Hachette UK's policy is to use papers that are natural, renewable and recyclable products and made from wood grown in sustainable forests. The logging and manufacturing processes are expected to conform to the environmental regulations of the country of origin.

Contents

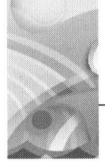

Introduction

About this guide

This unit guide is the third in a series of four that covers the whole Edexcel specification for AS and A-level physical education. Its aim is to help you prepare for the Unit 3 examination by providing an understanding of the key concepts, as well as looking at revision strategies and examination techniques. It is divided into three sections:

- **Introduction** — this provides advice on how to use the guide, an explanation of the skills required in A2 PE and suggestions for effective revision. It also offers assistance and guidance on how to apply your knowledge in the examination.
- **Content Guidance** — this summarises the specification content of Unit 3.
- **Questions and Answers** — this contains mock questions for you to try, together with sample answers to the questions and examiner's comments on how these answers could be improved. Each question has been attempted by two candidates, Candidate A and Candidate B. Their answers, along with the examiner's comments, should help you to see what you need to do to score a good grade. They also demonstrate how you can easily miss marks even though you may understand the topic.

Content Guidance

The specification content is divided into three sections. The first examines short-term preparation for optimum sports performance; the second looks at long-term preparation; the third focuses on the management of elite performance.

Short-term preparation

The section further divides short-term preparation into the physiological, psychological and technological roles involved in achieving optimum performance. Key concepts include:

- the basic principles involved in warming up, i.e. how, why and what is done and the benefits gained
- the role of energy manipulation in order to obtain and then maintain optimum performance
- the factors involved in acclimatisation and how athletes can overcome them in order to ensure that they perform optimally regardless of the environment
- the athlete's motivation and stress control in the short-term preparation phase
- strategies that can be used to help athletes and teams mentally prepare for competition
- external influences that can affect mental preparation in the short-term phase
- the selection of kit and equipment in the short-term preparation phase
- the use of ergogenic aids in short-term preparation
- the use of holding camps and pre-match rituals

- the effects of fatigue upon performance and how this can be delayed in order to maintain optimum performance for longer
- how athletes can best recover and the effects that this will have on subsequent performances

Long-term preparation

This section is divided into similar sections — physiological, psychological and techno-logical — while examining the long-term strategies that are available to elite performers who are attempting to achieve optimum performance. Key concepts include:

- the long-term effects of training upon the athlete, namely the physiological adapta-tions, which are related directly to the different methods of training
- the use of goal setting and mental training in long-term psychological training
- strategies that can help an athlete's self-development and tactics in long-term preparation
- mechanical issues in long-term technical preparation

Managing elite performance

Finally, this section investigates how elite athletes are supported throughout the world, looking at the history of support for elite sports, identifying the key stages of devel-opment and discussing the different types of support that different countries use. It also considers the benefits and issues relating to the use of sports institutes and acade-mies. Key concepts include:

- the different systems of elite support in various countries (the former East Germany, Australia, USA, UK)
- the needs of elite athletes in the twenty-first century
- the benefits of the academy model
- the role of technology in training analysis, enhancement and evaluation for sporting performance
- the concept of sports science and support

How should I use this guide?

The guide can be used throughout your physical education course — it is not *just* a revision aid. Because the Content Guidance is laid out in sections that correspond to those of the specification for Unit 3, you can use it:

- to check that your notes cover the material required by the specification
- to identify strengths and weaknesses
- as a reference for homework and internal tests
- during your revision to prepare 'bite-sized' chunks of related material, rather than being faced with a file full of notes

The Question and Answer section can be used to:

- identify the terms used by examiners in questions and what they expect of you
- familiarise yourself with the style of questions you can expect
- identify the ways in which marks are lost as well as the ways in which they are gained

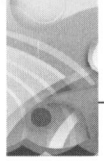

The specification

To make a good start to studying Unit 3, it is imperative that you have access to the unit specification. This can be obtained from your teacher or directly from the awarding body, Edexcel, at **www.edexcel.com**.

The specification identifies everything that needs to be covered and understood. It also informs you as to what could be in the final end-of-unit examination — if a topic is in the specification, then it could be examined; if it is not, it will not be examined.

Study skills and revision strategies

Revision and preparation for examinations are highly personal. However, there are common approaches that should be employed by all. Being successful in any subject depends on:

- **understanding** — the ability to follow a particular concept
- **learning** — the ability to recall the concept without prompts
- **application** — the ability to use the knowledge you have learnt to answer the questions that have been asked

The Question and Answer section of this guide deals with application.

Past papers can be useful. They will familiarise you with the format of the questions and the language used. There are also mark schemes and examiner's reports available. These indicate the sorts of mistakes made by students when faced with particular questions. They also include some model answers.

There are several ways of learning and individuals will have particular favourites determined by their preferred learning style(s), whether it is auditory, visual or kinaesthetic. However, there are common areas of good practice that could and should be adopted by all students. Whatever your preferred style, you must work out a revision plan.

What you must do

- Leave yourself enough time to cover *all* the material identified in the specification for Unit 3.
- Make sure that you actually have all the material to hand (use this book as a basis).
- Identify weaknesses early in your preparation so that you have time to do something about them.
- Familiarise yourself with the terminology used in the examination questions (see p. 7).

Things you could do to help you learn

- Copy selected sections of your notes.
- Summarise your notes into a more compact format, including the key points.

- Create your own flash cards — write key points on postcards (carry them around with you for quick revision during a coffee break or on the bus).
- Make audio recordings of your notes and/or the key points and play these back.
- Make a PowerPoint presentation of the key points and use this to revise in the last few days before the unit test.
- Discuss a topic with a friend who is studying the same course.
- Try to explain a topic to someone who is *not* following the course.
- Practice examination questions on a topic.

Approaching the unit examination

Terms used in examination questions

You will be asked precise questions in the examination so you can save a lot of valuable time — as well as ensuring you score as many marks as possible — by knowing what is expected. Terms most commonly used are explained below.

Brief

This means that only a short statement of the main points is needed.

Define

This requires you to state the meaning of a term, without using the term itself.

Describe

This is a request for factual detail about a structure or process, expressed logically and concisely, without explanation.

Discuss

You are required to give a critical account of various viewpoints and arguments on the topic set, drawing attention to their relative importance and significance.

Evaluate

This means that a judgement of evidence and/or arguments is required.

Explain

This means that reasons have to be given in your answer.

Identify

This requires a word, phrase or brief statement to show that you recognise a concept or a theory in an item.

List

This requires a sequence of numbered points one below the other, with no further explanation.

Outline

This means giving only the main points, i.e. don't go into detail. Don't be tempted to write more than necessary — this will waste time.

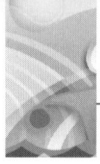

State

A brief concise answer, with no reasons, is required.

Suggest

This means that the question has no fixed answer and a wide range of reasonable responses is acceptable.

What is meant by...?

This usually requires a definition. The amount of information needed is indicated by the mark allocation.

The unit examination

When you finally open the test paper, it can be quite a stressful moment. Remember that you must answer *all* the questions on the paper. Read each one carefully and allocate the marks in your mind. Simply writing about the topic referred to in the question will not be enough — you must answer the question.

Some other strategies include:
- *do not* begin to write as soon as you open the paper
- *do* read the questions thoroughly before you start your answers
- *do* identify those questions about which you feel most confident
- *do* answer *first* those questions about which you feel most confident regardless of order in the paper
- *do* read the question carefully — if you are asked to explain, then explain, don't just describe
- *do* take notice of the mark allocation and try to match this to the number of points you make in your answer
- *do* try to stick to the point in your answer

Time allocation

Do not waste time writing things that will not get you marks! For example:

Outline the reasons why an athlete would complete a warm-up prior to exercise.

(2 marks)

This is a straightforward question. When it appeared in an examination paper most students scored the full 2 marks. Many students, however, scored those marks in a couple of sentences and then wasted time writing another half page. Remember, 2 marks means you have to make just two points.

Break the question down

Ask yourself, 'How many things am I being asked to do?' Identify the different parts of the question to ensure that you do everything asked, therefore making it possible to gain all of the marks available. Take the following example:

Identify and explain the stages of a warm-up for a sport of your choice. (6 marks)

This question had 3 marks available for the first part of the question — *identifying* the stages of a warm-up — and 3 marks for the second part of the question — *explaining* the stages of a warm-up.

Plan your answer

Try to be concise, but make sure that you include enough points to match the marks available. Take the following example:

Identify three additional responses to exercise. Explain why each occurs and the benefit provided for the performer. (9 marks)

This question asks you to:
- identify
- explain why
- state the benefits

It would be easy to write a mini-essay that contains a lot of detailed sports science, but fails to answer one or more parts of the question. The question asks for three things, three times. By structuring your answer, you should be able to identify nine points:
- first response
- explain why this response occurs
- state the benefit from this response
- second response
- explain why the second response occurs...and so on

Answer the question set

It is important to answer the question set and not the question that you wish had been set. For example:

Identify the adaptations to, and benefits for, the muscular system that result from aerobic training. (3 marks)

Answers relating to the cardiovascular or skeletal systems will waste time and not score any marks.

If questions ask specifically for examples, you must include them in your answers. In many questions, if you do not give any examples, you may not gain any marks.

Content Guidance

This section is a guide to **Unit 3: Preparation for Optimum Sports Performance**. The main areas covered are:

- short-term strategies that can help to ensure that optimum performance is achieved
- long-term strategies that can help to ensure that optimum performance is achieved
- how, once achieved, elite performance can be managed

Short-term preparation

Short-term physiological preparation

Key points
- **The warm-up** — what it is, why it is undertaken, how it is undertaken in terms of the stages to be performed and the benefits achieved.
- **Stretching** — different types of stretches, how they are performed and the benefits achieved.
- **Sources of energy for exercise** — what energy is, the different types of energy available to an athlete and strategies of short-term dietary manipulation.
- **Short-term acclimatisation** — what this includes, the extent to which the environment can affect performance and also the extent to which the athlete can minimise this effect.

The warm-up

Warm-up has become a generic term used to describe the activities performed in preparation for a sporting event. As such, the fundamental objective of a warm-up is to fully prepare the athlete both mentally and physically. By completing a warm-up, the athlete should enjoy an improved performance and also reduce the likelihood of injury.

The body functions optimally at a specific temperature. Extremes of temperature will adversely affect performance. As a result, during the warm-up, core and localised temperatures should be increased to reach that optimum temperature. At the same time, the body will begin to employ a more efficient system of temperature regulation.

Many of the physiological aspects of a warm-up can and should be targeted to the specific activity being performed. For example, if a ball is used in the activity then it should be incorporated into the warm-up. Therefore, completion of a warm-up can also improve the neuromuscular aspects of a performance.

Warm-up stages
There are three accepted stages of a warm-up, with the final stage often being divided to create an additional stage:
(1) **Initial preparation** involves gross motor activities that are designed, among other things, to increase the core body temperature, increase localised muscular temperature and increase rates of circulation and ventilation.
(2) **Injury prevention** involves mobility exercises — often including different types of stretches — to increase joint mobility and also muscle elasticity. In total, this will increase localised flexibility.

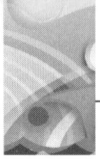

(3) Skills practice involves performing skills or aspects of skills in isolation and at a lower intensity than would be expected during the performance.

(4) Sports specific (either as an extension of skills practice or as a separate stage of the warm-up) involves skills or combinations of skills being performed as they would be within the performance in terms of intensity and competition.

Stage	Title	Aim	How achieved	Benefits
1	Initial preparation	Encourage the necessary responses to facilitate improved performance	Gross motor skills Slow continuous exercise, increasing in intensity	• Release of adrenaline = increase in heart rate • Increase in ventilation, speeding up of oxygen delivery • Heat generation • Speeds up localised muscular metabolism • Dilation of capillaries • Increased muscle elasticity = greater force and speed of contraction • Decreased muscle viscosity = greater force and speed of contraction • Reduced viscosity of the muscles = greater flexibility
2	Injury prevention	Minimise the risk of injury	Stretching (static, passive, ballistic, dynamic, PNF)	• Less risk of injury • Improves the tension/tone over a greater range of movement • Enables a greater force to be exerted • Reduces loss of performance with age • Assists in postural improvements
3	Skills practice	Strengthen mind–muscle link Improve confidence	Partner/group practice	• Improved reaction and responses due to increased speed of nerve impulses • Improved timing for skills = minimising risk of injury
4	Sport specific	Final preparation for the 'live' performance	Partner/group practice with an increased intensity/ simulation of 'performance' conditions	• Simulates the actual performance, thus completing the preparatory stage to the appropriate level • Develops confidence • Aids performance

Tip Make sure that you can explain how to carry out a warm-up, the reasons for undertaking one and the benefits achieved as a result of the warm-up activities performed.

Types of stretching

Stretching is an excellent way of increasing muscle elasticity. Muscle elasticity and joint structure are the two determinants of localised flexibility — the greater the flexibility, the greater the potential for movement but also for improved efficiency of movement.

Pre-activity stretching is a topical subject. Debates exist as to its benefits in terms of injury prevention and it is difficult to measure the effectiveness of pre-exercise stretching in this regard. Stretching is certainly the best way of maintaining or improving muscle elasticity. Performing stretching during a cool down is an excellent way of maintaining elasticity while aiding recovery. Performing static stretching in preparation for more sport-specific stretching during a warm-up is almost certainly good practice. However, whether there are benefits to be gained from performing a few static stretches before embarking upon a particularly ballistic activity, such as trampolining or high hurdling, is debatable. Overall, the main concern within any pre-exercise routine is to ensure that nothing is carried out that would be detrimental to safety and performance.

The different modes of stretching are
- **Static** — the muscle is taken to its limit and held under tension.
- **Ballistic** — momentum is used to force the fibres to stretch over a greater range.
- **PNF (proprioceptive neuromuscular facilitation)** — the muscle is stretched to its limit and then performs an isometric contraction while stretched. Relax and repeat.
- **Active stretching** — the performer stretches the body part.
- **Passive stretching** — the performer allows a partner or object to perform the stretch.
- **Dynamic** — the muscle is stretched through a range of motion/movement.

Intensity and duration
The **intensity** and **duration** of a warm-up are dependent upon a combination of factors, but on the whole will vary according to:
- the type of performance/activity to be performed
- the environment in which it is to be performed
- the person completing the performance

A warm-up should be designed to prepare the athlete for a specific performance/activity and to ensure that performance is at an optimum level. For example, if the activity will involve working at an anaerobic threshold then the warm-up must also go into this zone. This will prepare the body so that it is better able to cope with the increased heat and build up of lactic acid that will inevitably occur during the actual performance.

If the activity is being performed in cold or hot conditions then this too will have a bearing on the intensity and duration of the warm-up. A cold day will require a longer warm-up period, with a lower than usual starting intensity that is increased over a period of time. By contrast, a marathon runner about to compete in hot and humid conditions will be conscious of not wanting to overheat (requiring thermoregulation) and also of the need to remain hydrated. A shorter warm-up, involving low-intensity activity with bouts of short, high-intensity intervals is required. This will be sufficient to prepare the athlete but not overheat or dehydrate their body.

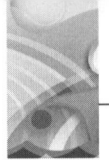

Consequently all warm-ups will need to be individual and specific to both the individual and also the performance to follow.

Sources of energy for exercise

A **balanced diet** contains appropriate quantities of all of the food groups and ensures that calories in do not exceed calories out. There are seven food groups, as shown in the table below, each of which performs a vital function for the body.

	Food group	Main bodily function	Good source of the food group
Energy providers	Carbohydrates	High-intensity fuel. Aids the utilisation of fats as an energy source. There are two types of carbohydrate: simple and complex.	Foods containing sugars and starch, e.g. fruit, pasta, wheat, cereals, chocolate
	Fats	Low-intensity energy. Insulation. There are two types of fat: soluble and insoluble.	Fish, animal and dairy products
	Proteins	Growth, repair and 'last resort' energy. Proteins are made from amino acids of which there are two types: essential and non-essential.	Meats, soya, dairy products
Non energy providers	Vitamins	Required to facilitate physiological functions. There are two main groups of vitamin: fat-soluble and water-soluble.	Animal and dairy products, fruits, vegetables and grains
	Minerals	Aid vitamin absorption. Provide the structure for things such as bones and teeth, and are essential in many bodily functions. Major minerals include: calcium, magnesium, potassium and sodium. Trace minerals include: zinc and fluorine.	Vegetables, fruits, fish, nuts
	Fibre	Essential for healthy bowel function. There are no calories, vitamins or minerals in fibre and it is not digested when eaten. There are two types of fibre: soluble and insoluble.	Plant foods, e.g. fruit, vegetables, beans and oats
	Water	Involved in almost every bodily function. Primarily seen in its role during thermoregulation and transport.	Fruits and water as a drink

As you can see from the table, three of the seven food groups can provide the body with energy: carbohydrates, fats and proteins. Each is used by the body at different times and to provide different types of energy.

For an athlete, carbohydrates will be the primary food that is eaten with consideration for performance or training. There are two types of carbohydrate: simple and complex. Simple carbohydrates have a simple structure that can be quickly and easily broken down into the basic glucose unit and so enter the blood. Complex carbohydrates have a more complex structure that takes longer to break down into glucose and enter the blood.

When performing above a certain intensity level — and that level will be different for every individual — the body does not have sufficient time to make the required energy from fats. Consequently it will use carbohydrates as its main energy source. The body stores carbohydrates within the body in a structure called **glycogen**. This is similar in structure to complex carbohydrate. The body has approximately 90 minutes of muscle glycogen available if all stores are full. However, that time level is dependent on the intensity at which an activity is performed. The greater the intensity, the quicker the levels of muscle glycogen are depleted. So if a performance is to last for 90 minutes or longer, and if the performance is likely to be competitive, then the athlete needs to give serious consideration to their energy supplies.

Tip Make sure that you know the types of energy available to a performer both before and during an event, and also how these might differ as a result of climate, duration and intensity of the event.

Dietary manipulation describes the practice of altering an athlete's food and drink intake to take into account the requirements of their event or performance. For example, an athlete can supplement their glycogen levels during performance by eating or drinking energy gels, bars or drinks.

In order to successfully target dietary manipulation, consideration must be taken of the rate at which the athlete is expending energy and the rate at which they can consume it. A person can digest approximately 1 gram of carbohydrate per kilogram of body weight per hour during a performance. Consequently, an 80 kg athlete can only digest 80 g of carbohydrates per hour. However, they could quite easily be burning in excess of 600 calories per hour, which would equate to 150 g of carbohydrates. With such a high number of calories being used, supplementation during a long-distance event will not *prevent* the depletion of muscle glycogen and blood glucose — it will only delay it. The solution is to condition the athlete's body to burn fat at a higher intensity of exercise, therefore conserving muscle glycogen and blood glucose stores. Carbohydrate loading offers this solution.

Carbohydrate loading

The theory behind carbohydrate loading, or carbo-loading, is quite simple. As we saw above, muscle glycogen (which is similar to complex carbohydrate) is the energy used by the body for high-intensity activity. The body has a limit of approximately 90

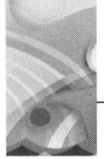

minutes' worth of muscle glycogen. If an event lasts in excess of 90 minutes then there will be insufficient energy. If an athlete can increase their body's stores of muscle glycogen then they can exercise harder and for longer.

However, simply increasing the athlete's carbohydrate input would just result in the excess being converted into fat. In order to make a body adapt and want to store more muscle glycogen, it must be encouraged to do so. This is done by following the super-compensation principle shown in the graph below.

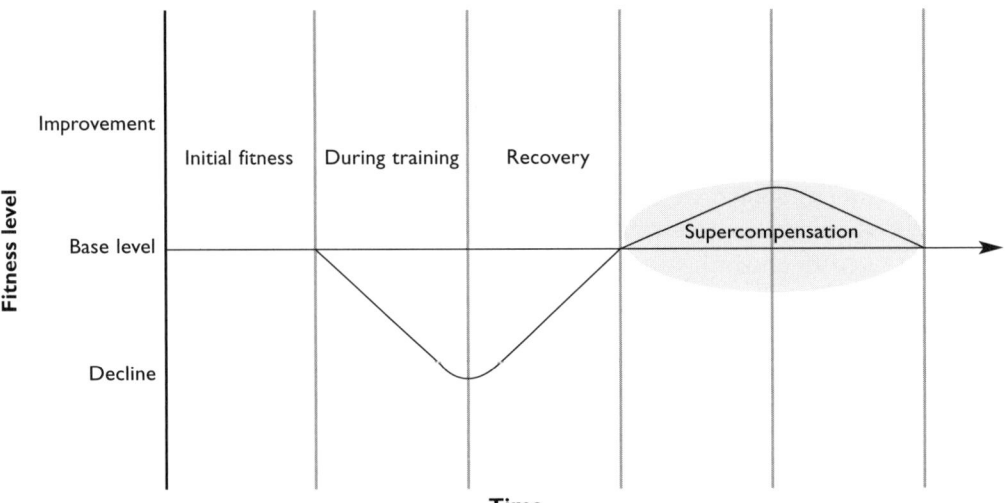

The supercompensation principle

For the body to want to increase its muscle glycogen stores it must be stressed into doing so. Firstly, the athlete needs to deplete the current muscle glycogen stores, as is usual during training and performance. Then, rather than eating to replenish the stores, they are maintained at a near depleted state. This will stress the body and when full levels of carbohydrate are once again available it will seek to hold on to more.

Hydration

Hydration is a term used to describe the state the body is in when it has optimal water content. **Dehydration** is when water content is low to the point where it is beginning to affect the functioning and efficiency of the body. Water is essential in order for the body to function. Every physiological process within the body requires water and almost two-thirds of our bodies are made up of water.

Losing water

The body loses water in a variety of ways:

- through daily urine output
- through sweating — the hotter the climate or the greater the intensity or duration of activity, the more a person will sweat

- through the act of respiration
- through ventilation as air has to be moistened as it enters the body

The adverse effect of dehydration on performance can be seen in the table below.

% body weight lost as sweat during a performance	Effect of water loss upon performance
1%	Loss of 5%
2%	Loss of 10%
4%	Loss of 25%
5%	Potential failure to complete
Greater than 5%	Potentially fatal

Creatine loading

Creatine is produced naturally in the body and helps to supply energy to muscle nerve cells. It is converted to and from phosphocreatine by the enzyme creatine kinase. The benefits of creatine as a dietary supplement are somewhat disputed, although many international athletes have undertaken creatine loading. The benefits claimed from creatine loading are an increase in lean muscle mass (and consequently high-intensity power) and an increased proportion of phosphocreatine within the muscle (making high-intensity energy last for longer and recovery faster). There is some evidence that taking creatine supplements can marginally increase athletic performance for high-intensity anaerobic cycling sprinters. However, benefits for swimmers or distance runners have been less evident.

Dietary requirements for exercise: a summary

A balanced diet helps to maintain general health. Any activity or change to the norm will require that a diet is modified to take the changes into account. By looking at the role of each of the seven food groups and by analysing an athlete's activity (for example, what type of fuel is required for training, for performing, in order to adapt, what level of water and electrolytes need to be replaced), it is possible to plan a diet to maximise sporting performance.

Short-term acclimatisation

To prepare for differences in environmental conditions, individuals and teams will go through a period of acclimatisation when preparing for global sports competitions. It can take between five and ten days for a performer to acclimatise (respond and adapt) to changes in heat and humidity.

Optimum sports performance means that everything must be functioning as well as possible. Training for 12 months for a major event becomes pointless if the immediate factors of the local environment are not properly considered. Factors such as high or

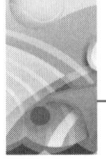

low temperature, prevailing wind, a wet or even dry surface, humidity, altitude and pollution, can all affect performance dramatically.

Heat adaptation

When an athlete performs in conditions that are different to those with which they are familiar, a variety of factors will need to be considered:

- Hot and humid conditions make it difficult to lose heat and therefore significantly increase the likelihood of heat exhaustion.
- Hot and dry conditions will increase the level of water lost through sweat and therefore increase the likelihood of dehydration, leading to heat exhaustion.
- Cold conditions necessitate more clothing which in turn leads to increased sweating and greater potential for dehydration.

These different climatic conditions mean that hydration planning strategies need to be implemented over and above those that are implemented during normal exercise conditions. For example, in order to acclimatise fully to increased heat, the body will require between 8–14 days during which low-intensity exercise is performed while consuming upwards of 8 litres of additional water. Surprisingly, consuming excess water and electrolytes does not speed up the process of heat acclimatisation.

Increased plasma volume

While undergoing heat acclimatisation, the athlete might experience a temporary increase in blood plasma volume. This is as a result of an increased production of plasma proteins added to the increased concentration of electrolytes that are taken with water in order to aid hydration. This increase is likely during the first five days of exercise in heat exposure but is temporary — levels will revert to normal after between 8 and 14 days.

Effects of altitude

The reduced partial pressure of oxygen at altitude makes it difficult for the body to inspire as much oxygen per breath as it can at sea level. This means that the athlete will experience a hypoxic state at a lower intensity, which effectively lowers their VO_2max and their anaerobic threshold. As a result, performance of any aerobic activity at an altitude where the partial pressure of oxygen is lower than 20 kPa is likely to deteriorate.

Acclimatisation can be undertaken for altitude. This involves a period of approximately 14 days at altitude. Initially, exercise will be at a lower intensity than the athlete's norm. However, as the body adapts the intensity can be increased. Athletes likely to have to perform at altitude should ensure that they have undertaken sufficient acclimatisation. Many endurance athletes deliberately train at altitude — altitude training — in an attempt to improve their aerobic efficiency. The theory is that if an athlete can perform at altitude then performance will be improved on returning to sea level, where there is more oxygen available.

Tip Make sure that you can explain how different environments can affect performance and how athletes can overcome these effects, via acclimatisation, in order to maintain their perform levels.

Short-term psychological preparation

Key points

- **Motivation and stress control** — the effects of these during short-term preparation for sport.
- **Strategies** to aid mental short-term preparation.
- **External influences** — what these are and how they can affect a performer's short-term psychological preparation.

This section considers how performers can prepare mentally for sport in the last few hours before competition. It looks at the factors that affect mental preparation and identifies some of the training and strategies that can be used to ensure a competitor performs at their optimum level.

Sports psychology is the application of the science of behaviour to exercise and sports participation. Elite performers and their coaches use sports psychology to help them gain a competitive edge. A knowledge of sports psychology, or the intervention of a sports psychologist, can help performers to manage their stress and anxiety more effectively, improving their concentration and motivation.

Successful performers in sport tend to have:
- high levels of self-confidence
- a task-oriented focus
- control over their anxiety levels
- determination and commitment

Motivation and stress control

In sport, the drive to play well is referred to as **motivation**. Motivation can be influenced by many factors, which in turn can lead to a performer experiencing anxiety. In short-term preparation, coaches and players use strategies to ensure that the motivation of their performers is at its optimum level.

One factor influencing motivation is **self-confidence**, though the impact of this may depend on the experience of the performer. For beginners, a lack of self-confidence will mean that they feel they are going to perform badly. For elite performers, a lack of self-confidence is usually related to specific situations or venues.

Bandura's (1977) theory of self-efficacy suggests that self-confidence is often specific to a particular situation. Bandura states that a performer's self-efficacy is influenced by four factors:
- **Performance accomplishments** — if a performer has been successful in the past, then feelings of self-confidence are likely to be high.
- **Vicarious experiences** — if a performer watches others perform and achieve success, then they are likely to experience high self-efficacy.

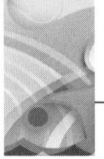

- **Verbal persuasion** — when significant others can encourage and support a performer, then self-confidence will be high.
- **Emotional arousal** — how a performer feels about their level of arousal can affect their confidence level.

Anxiety and arousal

Anxiety is a natural reaction to threat in the environment — part of our preparation for flight or fight. Anxiety in sport has three dimensions:
- **cognitive** — worry and negative feelings about a performance
- **somatic** — physiological symptoms, such as raised heart rate, increased perspiration, shortness of breath
- **behavioural** — experiencing tension, agitation and restlessness

In sport, performers can suffer from two types of anxiety:
- **State anxiety** is situation specific and can be linked to a particular role (such as penalty taking), place, or level of competition.
- **Trait anxiety** is a general and enduring feeling of apprehension.

The concept of anxiety is closely linked to **arousal** — a state of alertness. Arousal is usually displayed on a continuum from low (for example when sleeping) to high (for example when experiencing intense excitement). In sport, the aim is to be in a state of high arousal.

> **Tip** Make sure that you can define 'trait anxiety' and 'state anxiety'.

Effects on performance

In sport, the level of arousal can have either a positive or negative effect on performance. Jones and Swain (1992) state that most elite athletes view pre-competition arousal as a positive feeling of alertness, rather than as anxiety, whereas novice or less-experienced athletes have a negative response to this rise in arousal. There are four main theories that link arousal and anxiety with performance:
- The **inverted-U hypothesis**, developed by **Yearkes and Dodson** (1908). This suggests that as arousal increases, so does performance, but only up to a certain level. Beyond this level, further increases in arousal will cause a reduction in performance.
- **Drive theory**, developed by **Hull** (1943). This suggests a proportional linear relationship between arousal and performance. The higher a sports performer's arousal, the better the performance.
- The **catastrophe model**, developed by **Hardy** (1996). This suggests that arousal has different effects on sports performance depending on cognitive anxiety. Arousal will increase performance when cognitive anxiety is low, but may lead to a sudden catastrophic decline in performance when cognitive anxiety is relatively high.
- The **processing efficiency theory**, developed by **Eysenck and Calva** (1992). This suggests that anxiety may affect processing efficiency rather than task effectiveness.

When an athlete cannot cope with an increase in anxiety, they may **choke**. Choking in sport is defined as an athlete's inability to perform at their optimum level and can result in the sudden impairment or failure of sports performance. The potential for choking depends on both the athlete and the situation. Choking usually occurs when an athlete is overly concerned about what others (team mates, coaches or an audience) think about their performance.

Tip Make sure you can define 'choking'.

Strategies to prevent anxiety and choking
- Set achievable goals. Performance review monitoring (PMR) involves setting goals and identifying areas that need further work, so that athletes and coaches track progress regularly.
- Use imagery before a competition to review strategy and technique and create a sense of confidence. Imagery (also known as visualisation) means creating a series of mental pictures, and is used by performers to improve their concentration and promote feelings of self-confidence.
- Use positive self-talk, both in preparation and in competition. Self-talk can be used in conjunction with specific skills to help an athlete focus on correct technique. For example, a rugby player could use the phrase 'low and drive' before tackling an opponent.
- Use cue utilisation. The performer's attention level can be enhanced by concentrating on the cues that are most relevant.
- Practise relaxation exercises to help with the symptoms of somatic anxiety.
  - Self-directed relaxation is when the performer concentrates on each of their muscle groups separately and relaxes them.
  - Progressive relaxation training involves a performer feeling the tension in their muscles and getting rid of this tension by 'letting go'.
- Use music prior to a competition to help maintain focus by controlling negative thoughts.

Aggression versus assertion
Aggression (although it is a term sometimes loosely used in sport) means 'intent to harm outside the laws of the game'. It can have either a positive or a negative effect on performance. When aggression is controlled or channelled it becomes **assertion** and it is this concept that should be encouraged in sport.

There are two key theories that are used to explain the occurrence of aggression in sport:
- The **instinct theory** suggests that aggression is an innate biological drive and that sport simply gives it an outlet. The frustration–aggression hypothesis (a version of drive theory) states that blocking goals can cause frustration, which then leads to aggression.
- The **social learning theory** developed by Bandura states that people learn to be aggressive by watching others.

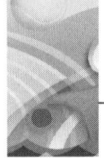

Strategies to reduce aggression
- Internal control of arousal levels
- Punishment of aggressive acts
- Positive reinforcement of non-aggressive behaviour

External influences
There are a number of external influences that can affect a performer's preparation for sport in the short-term phase.

Home advantage
Studies on the concept of home advantage suggest that teams playing at home win, on average, 56–64% of their matches. This advantage is especially relevant to indoor sports, a finding that may be linked to the so-called **proximity effect** — whereby crowds that are close to the action (as in basketball) are said to increase the audience's influence.

Social facilitation
Social facilitation refers to the influence other people can have on performance. These other people may include:
- **co-actors** other participants (team mates and opponents)
- **audience** — spectators
- **significant others** — family, coaches

These people may have a facilitating (positive) or inhibiting (negative) effect on performance.

There are a number of theories that are used to explain social facilitation:
- **Triplett** (1898). His findings, published in the *American Journal of Psychology* (9: 507–33), showed that cyclists' performance increased by 30% when they were riding in a group of other cyclists. Other research has since confirmed that the presence of others tends to result in an increased level of performance.
- **Ringlemann** (1913) — the **Ringlemann effect.** His findings showed that the increase in performance only occurred up to a certain number of co-actors. When group size gets too big, there is a tendency for some in the group to lose motivation and rely on others — this is known as **social loafing**.
- **Zajonc** (1965). He developed the drive theory to explain the link between arousal and performance. Drive theory suggests that our learned behaviours tend to be our **dominant responses**.

Strategies to help performers cope with crowds
- Practise selective attention to help cut out the awareness of others.
- Use cognitive visualisation techniques and strategies, such as imagery/mental rehearsal, to help focus on the task.
- Ensure essential skills are over-learned to ensure that the dominant response is successful.

- Use evaluative practices. Performers are encouraged to give feedback on each other's performance.
- Practise with simulated crowd noises using audio recordings.
- Incorporate stress management and relaxation techniques into training.

Evaluation apprehension

Cottrell (1972) studied the concept of social facilitation and concluded that the key influence on performance was not simply the presence of others, but whether the performer felt the audience was judging or evaluating the performance. This is called **evaluation apprehension** and leads to arousal and the resulting dominant response.

Importance of competition

The more important the level of competition, generally the higher the level of state anxiety the performer will experience. Most of this pressure and anxiety will come from external sources — the bigger the competition, the more the media, audience and significant others will talk and project the result. Again, it is the way the performer perceives this extra pressure that is the key to controlling the anxiety. A cup final or international fixture will heighten the stakes, and there is a chance that the participants will feel less confident.

This concept was developed by Martens into the theory of **competitive anxiety**. Competitive anxiety can be defined as an individual's tendency to perceive competitive situations as threatening and to respond to these situations by experiencing state anxiety.

Environmental factors

In terms of anxiety, the effect of the environment depends not so much on the playing field or physical setting, but rather on the people in that setting. The social environment could include the crowd, other competitors (including team mates and opponents), coaches, and in elite sport the media in its various forms.

Novice performers perform best in low-arousal environments. The low-arousal environment would be where no-one is watching or evaluating the performance, and where the importance of competition is low.

The nature of the audience can also have an effect on performance. If the crowd is noisy and aggressive then the performer may feel more anxious and may also become more aggressive themselves. The proximity of the crowd can also influence performance — if the crowd is close to the court or pitch, the performer may feel threatened, which may cause their level of anxiety to increase. Conversely, some performers may feel reassured by a supportive crowd close to the action.

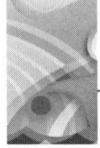

Short-term technical preparation

Key points

- **Kit and equipment** — explain their use in the short-term preparation phase.
- **Ergogenic aids** — explain and describe their use for short-term preparation in sport.
- **Drugs and supplements** — discuss their use in sport.
- **Pre-match holding camps and pre-performance rituals** — explain the reasons for their use.

You need to be able to discuss the factors that athletes consider in their short-term technical preparation for sport. Short-term preparation refers to the time immediately before competition. This may be restricted to a few hours, but normally in elite sport the build-up to a global sports competition can begin several days before the event.

Kit and equipment

Most elite teams have specialist kit managers who help performers with their technical preparation. Technical sports, such as skiing, cycling and sailing, often involve large teams of people and a great deal of kit and equipment to enable adjustment to the performance conditions.

Factors that affect the selection of playing kit and equipment include:
- climate, including temperature, humidity and wind
- playing surface, for example choice of footwear or length of studs
- indoor or outdoor, for example whether a stadium roof is closed or open (when the roof is closed, the atmosphere is more humid, so shirts made from a lighter fabric are used)
- protection/reducing injury, for example wearing shoulder pads in rugby or kneepads in volleyball

The climate can have a major impact on physical performance. Players need to wear kit that helps them maintain a constant core temperature. Many players now wear compression clothing underneath their playing equipment. Those performing in warm environments favour lightweight fabrics.

In some sports, air or fluid dynamics can influence performance. Teams and performers will select clothing or other strategies specifically designed to reduce this effect. Traditionally in swimming and cycling, performers 'shave down' in preparation for competition, but whether this has any real impact on performance is debatable — it may be more of a ritual, helping the performer to prepare mentally for competition. In sports such as sprinting and swimming, many performers use aerodynamic suits in an attempt to reduce drag and improve their speed and power.

Use of ergogenic aids

Ergogenic aids are substances or devices that enhance energy production, use or recovery, and provide athletes with a competitive advantage. With the margins of winning and losing in global sport being so small, teams and performers are constantly looking for the competitive edge that will give them this small percentage improvement.

> **Tip** Make sure that you can define 'ergogenic aid'.

There are so many ergogenic aids available to athletes that it is useful to group them under the following headings:

- **Mechanical aids** — these include simple technologies, such as heart-rate monitors used to identify training thresholds, or more complex systems, such as hypoxic chambers. (See the notes on ice vests and cycle ergs below.)
- **Chemical aids** — these may be naturally occurring products, such as ginseng, which has been used as a supplement, or chemical copies, such as creatine monohydrate. (See the notes on drugs and supplements below.)
- **Physiological aids** — techniques such as acupuncture and sports massage.
- **Psychological aids** — such as the use of imagery, music and hypnosis.

Mechanical aids

Ice vests and thermoregulation

It is usual for the Olympic Games and most world cup tournaments to be held in the summer months. When body temperature rises, the blood is diverted away from the muscle to the skin in an attempt to cool down. This means less blood flows to the muscle, which has a negative effect on performance. Therefore, performers need to plan and use technology to help them control their body temperature. Companies such as Nike have developed ice vests or cooling vests that can help athletes to stabilise their temperature.

Cycle ergo meters

Teams such as England Rugby use these static cycle machines on the edge of the pitch to allow substitutes to warm up and prepare better for entry into the game.

Chemical aids

Drugs and supplements in sport

Supplements are legal additions to an athlete's diet. They are legal because governing bodies of sport do not feel that their use is harmful to health. As more research is done, some supplements may in time become illegal drugs. **Dietary and nutritional supplements** are widely used in sport and are readily available on the high street. Most elite athletes take multi-vitamins and extra minerals in order to be able to recover from heavy workouts, as well as helping to prevent illness.

Drug-taking is the ultimate in sporting gamesmanship — breaking the rules in order to increase performance and the chances of winning. Athletes are known to take a range of performance-enhancing drugs. Most originated as genuine medical treatments, but their side effects have been used by athletes to improve their athletic

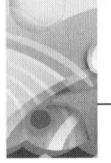

performance illegally. The range and availability of these types of drugs are constantly increasing, making control difficult.

The huge increase in rewards for winning means that the temptation to take drugs has become great for some athletes. According to the World Anti-Doping Code, there are three main factors that influence the legality of an ergogenic substance. A substance or practice is banned if it fulfils at least two of the following factors:
- physically enhances the performance of the athlete
- is detrimental to the athlete's health (some are potentially lethal)
- conflicts with the general spirit of sport

Major banned chemical ergogenic aids include:
- **stimulants** — amphetamine, cocaine, caffeine
- **diuretics** — furosemide, hydroclorothiazide
- **peptide hormones** — epogen, human growth hormone
- **beta blockers** — atenolol, labetolol
- **narcotic analgesics** — heroin, morphine
- **anabolic agents** — nandrolone, clenbuterol, androstenedione

The fine line between what is legal and illegal causes many dilemmas for both the performer and the authorities. A sprinter can legally take ginseng, although it contains substances that have advantageous effects. An athlete can train at high altitude to try to develop the efficiency of their blood system, but blood doping is illegal.

Pre-match camps

Pre-match camps are used as a base for training and preparation in the weeks and months before major competitions (see holding and preparation camps on p. 54).

Pre-match rituals

Many players and teams go through specific routines and programmes before they play. These routines help them to prepare physically and mentally for competition but, like any other aspect of preparation, need to be practised during the long-term training phase. The exact nature of these rituals will change depending on the sport and the individual but often they will include checking and preparing for many of the factors discussed above in the short-term preparation phase. An example of a ritual is the order in which players put on their kit — for example, putting on the left boot first.

Fatigue and the recovery process

Key points
- **Fatigue** — what fatigue actually represents and factors that bring it about. How an athlete can attempt to ensure that fatigue does not affect performance.
- **Recovery** — the timings and stages of recovery, what actually happens at any given

stage and how this can be encouraged. The benefits of speeding up recovery and the dangers of allowing it to take too long.

Causes of fatigue

Depletion of fuels

The body uses energy obtained from food to fuel movement. Carbohydrates, fats and proteins can provide the body with energy. When eaten, these food groups are broken down and the resulting **potential energy** is either sent to the muscles to be used or is stored. It can be stored in one of several forms and places:

- as adenosine triphosphate (ATP) in the muscle
- as phosphagencreatine (PC) in the muscle
- as muscle glycogen in the muscle
- as liver glycogen in the liver
- as body fat around the body

The body has two mechanisms — the **aerobic energy system** and the **anaerobic energy system** — that enable it to take stored potential energy and convert it into useable fuel (ATP). These two energy systems use three energy pathways:

- ATP-PC energy pathway (alactic energy pathway) — an anaerobic energy system
- lactic acid energy pathway — an anaerobic energy system
- aerobic energy pathway — an aerobic energy system

The body will use the appropriate energy system and pathway, taking stored energy from appropriate energy stores depending on the intensity of the activity being performed. See the table below to review the characteristics of the energy systems and pathways.

	ATP-PC energy pathway	Lactic acid energy pathway	Aerobic energy pathway
Energy taken from	Stored ATP and stored PC	Stored muscle glycogen	Stored muscle glycogen and body fat
Characteristics	• Instantly available • Supports maximal contractions/exercise intensity • Can sustain activity for 10–12 seconds only	• Quick to produce energy • Supports near maximal contractions/exercise intensity • Can sustain activity for between 60 seconds and 90 minutes depending on the intensity	• Complicated process means energy takes a little time to be produced • Can support submaximal exercise intensity • Can last almost indefinitely

When competing, speed is often a primary concern. The faster an athlete performs, the greater the amount of energy required and the faster the rate it is required at. The problem here is that people do not have a limitless supply of this type of energy.

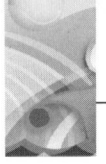

Consequently, the performer needs to compete at a level that manages energy supplies most efficiently. The balance is similar to that experienced by a Formula One racing driver. If he drives at the car's fastest speed throughout the entire race then the tyres and fuel will not last. Because of this, the car is driven at a little below maximum in order to complete the race.

Even when managing speed efficiently, there will be times when exercise intensity exceeds the available energy. When muscle glycogen levels begin to be depleted then the body will attempt to utilise glycogen stored in the liver. This poses an additional problem, however, as liver glycogen's primary role is that of providing neural energy. When liver glycogen levels begin to be depleted there will be low blood sugar levels, producing a feeling of lethargy and fatigue. Fat can then be metabolised if the intensity of the activity is low enough.

Waste product accumulation

Lactic acid is a by-product of metabolising glucose for energy and has historically been seen as a waste product that causes a burning sensation in the muscles. Lactic acid is produced when glucose is converted into ATP through the lactic acid energy pathway. Without the presence of oxygen to further break down the lactic acid, it builds up in the blood. When lactic acid measures 4 mmolls within the blood, it begins to build up more quickly than it can be utilised. This point is called the point of **onset of blood lactic acid accumulation** (OBLA).

However, rather than being a harmful waste product, scientists have now identified it as providing another fuel source for working muscles. It may still be responsible for the burning sensation experienced during intense exercise, but new research has confirmed that muscle cells can convert glucose or glycogen into lactic acid, which is absorbed into the mitochondria within the muscle cells where it is converted into a fuel. When training at a high intensity it is thought that the body creates additional proteins that help to absorb and convert lactic acid to energy.

Central governor theory

Researchers Tim Noakes and Alan St Clair Gibson developed a theory to challenge the conventional theory regarding muscle failure. They hypothesised that: 'Fatigue is an emotional response that begins in your brain, not a physiological one originating in the muscles!' Noakes and St Clair Gibson were initially intrigued about three issues:

- the role of lactic acid in the fatiguing process
- the number of muscle fibres recruited during progressively maximal intensity
- muscle glycogen depletion

The essence of their theory is the existence of a **central governor**. The brain paces the muscles to keep them back from the brink of exhaustion. When the brain decides it's time to quit, it creates the distressing sensations that are interpreted as muscle fatigue.

Dehydration and electrolyte loss

As we have already seen, dehydration is a state where the body contains below optimum water levels. The further into this state the body goes, the harder it is to operate efficiently and ultimately the more dangerous the state becomes. During exercise, the biggest cause of water loss is the body's attempts to cool itself — thermoregulation. During extreme endurance events, such as a marathon, up to 10% of water content can be lost. Water is lost through a variety of factors relating to exercise:

- during tissue respiration
- as a result of sweating — the amount of sweating is determined by external climate, body mass and metabolic rate (intensity)
- via greater quantities of air being expelled
- via the kidneys decreasing urine flow to try to prevent dehydration

As the body loses water it will also lose electrolytes, predominantly sodium and calcium. This has a number of effects that will lead to a loss of performance:

- decrease in the volume of plasma
- increase in blood viscosity, which will increase blood pressure
- impaired ability of the blood to carry and deliver oxygen
- impaired ability of the body to lose heat
- loss of efficiency and cramping of the muscles

Long term there will be a:

- decrease in blood pressure
- decrease in tissue fluid formation
- increased thirst
- increased heart rate

Recovery

Recovery begins as soon as exercise begins and it continues until the body has returned to a complete pre-exercise state. The body will start to replenish depleted stores, repair damaged tissue and remove waste. Although recovery during the first few hours can be split into two distinct stages, they do not happen one after the other but occur simultaneously.

Recovery during the first few hours
The slow component of recovery

This stage of recovery was originally thought to be concerned just with the removal of lactic acid. In reality, more is happening. The slow component is the vital anabolic phase during which the body repairs itself after the catabolic phase of exercise, be it training or performance. The quicker the body is able to recover, the sooner training can resume. The more training that an athlete can undertake, each session followed by full recovery, the greater the potential for improvement.

An active **cool down** can dramatically speed up the recovery phase. Just as the warm-up prepares for activity, the cool down should be seen as preparing for inactivity and also for the next training session. By gradually reducing the intensity of the activity over a period of approximately 20 minutes, the body is able to carry out the process of recovery much more effectively and quickly.

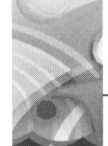

A cool down involves performing some kind of light, continuous exercise where the heart rate remains elevated. The purpose is to keep metabolic activity high, and capillaries dilated, so that oxygen can be flushed through the muscle tissue, removing and oxidising any lactic acid that remains. This will therefore prevent blood pooling in the veins, which can cause dizziness if exercise is stopped abruptly. The final part of the cool-down period should involve a period of stretching exercises.

Only once recovery has been completed should future training be considered.

Lactic acid utilisation during recovery

Lactic acid has been blamed for exercise-induced fatigue as well as post-exercise discomfort (see the section on DOMS below). However, as identified earlier, evidence is increasingly disputing both of these statements. For example, as much as half of all cardiac contractions are believed to be fuelled by a lactic acid energy substrate. The table below illustrates the percentage usage of lactic acid before it is removed by the body.

Destination	Approximate % of lactic acid involved
Oxidised into carbon dioxide and water	65
Converted into glycogen and then stored in muscle liver	20
Converted into protein	10
Converted into glucose	5

Restoration of ATP and PC — the fast component of recovery

The fast component of recovery is primarily concerned with the re-phosphorylisation of the muscles. When the body's supplies of muscle ATP and PC have been depleted, the body is vulnerable. Consequently, this element of recovery needs to take place quickly (see the table below).

Recovery time (seconds)	Muscle phosphagen restored (%)
10	10
30	50
60	75
90	87
120	93
150	97
180	99
210	101
240	102

As can be seen, this process takes place at a rapid rate. This explains why, when running a 1500 m race, an athlete can sprint at the beginning and recover sufficiently to be able to sprint once again by the end of the race.

Three mechanisms contribute to the regeneration of phosphocreatine:
- Energy from the aerobic conversion of carbohydrate into carbon dioxide and water is used to manufacture ATP from ADP and PC (the products of ATP consumption).
- Some of this ATP is immediately utilised to create PC using the following coupled reaction.

$$ATP \longrightarrow ADP + P_1 + energy$$
$$\downarrow$$
$$energy + P_1 + C \longrightarrow PC$$

- A small percentage of ATP, derived from lactic acid production, is made available for phosphagen replenishment.

EPOC

EPOC stands for **Excess Post-exercise Oxygen Consumption** and refers to the elevation of ventilation, temperature and heart rates after exercise when compared to levels before exercise began. During exhaustive exercise, for example, the body's temperature may increase by as much as 3 degrees. This increased body temperature will significantly speed up metabolic processes for some time post-exercise. All the processes that are needed in order to complete recovery require energy, and therefore oxygen. This is why the heart rate increases during recovery. Measuring heart rate, body temperature and ventilation rate can therefore give an indication of when recovery is complete.

Recovery processes requiring energy include:
- replenishing ATP stores, PC stores, muscle and liver glycogen stores
- tissue repair
- redistribution of calcium ions
- removal of carbon dioxide
- oxidisation of lactic acid
- reloading haemoglobin with oxygen — as much as 10% of recovery oxygen is directly used for this; a further 5% may be dissolved in the body's fluids and also used for this purpose
- the primary and secondary respiratory muscles will be working harder and will require more oxygen to do so
- the heart is also working harder and will require more oxygen

Recovery after 24 hours

DOMS

DOMS stands for **Delayed Onset Muscle Soreness** and refers to localised muscular soreness experienced after exercise has been completed. It is usually experienced 24 hours post-exercise and can last for anything up to 4 days in extreme cases.

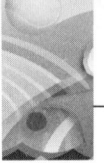

The soreness is caused as the body repairs muscle tissue that was damaged during the exercise. It must be noted that it is the *repair* of the tissue and not the initial damage that causes the muscle soreness. Damage to the muscle fibres is often associated with an excessive eccentric contraction — a rapid increase in intensity or a sudden change in the range of movement experienced during the exercise.

The potential for DOMS can be reduced by:
- gradually building up training intensity
- completing a thorough warm-up prior to exercise
- using cross training to expose the body to a variety of range of movements
- using aerobic training to increase capillarisation within the muscle, which allows faster saturation of the blood with oxygen and nutrients

Ergogenic aids to reduce fatigue and aid recovery

Compression clothing
The use of compression clothing, such as elastic shorts, tights and vests, has become increasingly widespread among athletes and fitness enthusiasts alike. Studies have confirmed that the use of such clothing gives better muscle alignment and structure, which reduces muscle damage, improves circulation, and increases awareness of muscle operation. This in turn leads to an increase in anaerobic threshold, power and endurance.

Research indicates that compression clothing material can reduce a performer's sweat rate by 30%. In addition, there is evidence to suggest that compression clothing may improve exercise performance by reducing the impact of hot and/or humid conditions on the body's thermoregulatory system.

Ice baths
It has been discovered that immersing parts of the body, or the whole body, in iced water can aid the recovery of athletes who have experienced high impact during their performance. Firstly, further damage to any torn fibres can be prevented through rapid constriction resulting from the sudden cold. Secondly, the body responds to the sudden cold by sending a significant blood rush to the immersed body parts. This helps to flush the damaged muscles, rapidly removing waste while also carrying oxygen and other beneficial nutrients.

Music
For many people, music provides a number of triggers: stimulation, invigoration, relaxation or meditation.

Tip Make sure that you can explain how fatigue can be delayed in order to maintain optimum performance for longer. You also need to know what can be done in order to speed up the recovery processes.

Long-term preparation

Long-term physiological preparation

The key to this section is to understand what you, as the performer, need to achieve from your training. What are the anatomical and physiological adaptations that would enhance your performance? Once this is understood, you need to plan how to achieve the required adaptations. What methods of training would best help you to achieve those adaptations?

Understanding adaptations

The term **adaptation** refers to a long-term and permanent change as a result of environmental factors. Training provides a stress for the body. Once this stress is experienced, the body will *respond* in order to manage the stress more effectively. An example of such a response would be an increase in heart rate. An increased heart rate is a temporary change — once the stress has finished, the heart rate reverts back to its normal rate. However, if the body experiences the same sort of stress, repeatedly, over a sustained period of time, then the body will make more permanent changes to help it cope. These could include an increase in the size of the heart. However, if the individual's environment changes again, say with a cessation of the regular stress — the exercise — then the body will once again adapt. In this case, the heart will atrophy, i.e. shrink in size.

> **Tip** Make sure that you can define 'adaptation'.

Anatomical adaptations (also known as structural adaptations) are changes to the structure of the body or body part. There are a limited number of anatomical adaptations that can occur. These include:

- change in size — larger or smaller
- change in number — more or less
- change in viscosity — thicker or thinner

Physiological adaptations are changes in function and are almost inevitably possible as a result of anatomical adaptations. For example, an increase in maximal cardiac output (Q), which is a physiological adaptation, will only be possible as a result of a larger cardiac chamber holding more blood, which is an anatomical or structural adaptation.

Methods of training

Aerobic and anaerobic

The terms aerobic and anaerobic are not methods of training as such, they are a reference to the mechanism used to produce energy. **Aerobic** means that energy is produced with oxygen. **Anaerobic** means that energy is being produced with

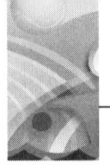

insufficient oxygen. When used in the context of training, aerobic training refers to any type of exercise that aims to stress the aerobic-producing capacity of the body, while anaerobic training is at a higher intensity and is designed to stress the body's capacity to work at that level.

The term 'threshold' is often used to describe the area between the two energy systems. The anaerobic threshold is where anaerobic systems begin to be the dominant energy providers.

Continuous training

Continuous training is performed at a constant work rate intensity — note that this refers to a constant *input*, such as heart rate, not a constant output, such as speed. This type of training is associated with long-duration, and therefore low- to medium-intensity, exercise. As such, it is used to stress the aerobic and endurance capabilities of the body.

Interval training

Interval training is based around a specific work to rest ratio (W:R), which is repeated. Training is performed for a specific amount of time, after which sufficient rest is allowed so that the body can recover, and then the training can be repeated. Because the work and rest periods can be adapted to suit the desired outcome (both in terms of intensity and duration), this type of training can be either aerobic or anaerobic in nature.

Plyometric training

Plyometric training is designed to stress the body's ability to work explosively. It exploits the elastic properties of muscles to develop power, coordination and dynamic balance. Muscles are preloaded by performing forced eccentric contractions that are immediately followed by concentric contractions. The force generated is considered to be greater than if a concentric contraction alone is performed. This is an anaerobic method of training.

Circuit/weight/resistance training

Circuit training involves different exercises being performed in sequence at exercise stations. The individual performs a number of repetitions or for a set amount of time before moving on to the next station. As with interval training, the intensity and duration of training can be manipulated to suit the individual and so circuit training can be either aerobic or anaerobic in nature. It can also be designed to improve flexibility or sport-specific skills.

Weight training involves working with a variable resistance that can be generated by the use of free weights or exercise machines. As the weight — which is the training intensity — is adaptable, this method of training is also adaptable. Although it is predominantly associated with anaerobic benefits, weight training can therefore also be used to develop localised muscular endurance.

Resistance training is similar to weight training, although the resistance is not necessarily variable. The individual can use body weight as the resistance, performing exercises such as sit-ups, press-ups, pull-ups, etc.

Speed training

Speed training is usually associated with maximum speed, and so is an anaerobic training method. Speed training can take the form of either maximal strength or maximal power training, as both are required for speed. It can also be in the form of 'over speed' training, such as downhill running or using elasticated belts and harnesses.

Fartlek training

Fartlek training is a variant of continuous training. Here, the training intensity is specifically changed during the course of the session. This type of training is performed with the idea of simulating performance or to temporarily stress the anaerobic functioning of the body before then encouraging the body to actively recover during a less intense phase of the training session.

Core stability training

Core stability refers to the target of the training rather than the type of training. The target is the muscles that make up the core of the body, such as the abdominal regions, obliques and erector spinae as well as muscles that work as synergists to gross motor movements. These muscles are required to be able to sustain work and so will be targeted with interval, circuit or resistance training.

SAQ (speed, agility, quickness)

SAQ will usually be performed at a high intensity, often within interval or circuit training, and will utilise equipment such as harnesses, ladders or similar obstacles.

Stretching

The different types of stretching were covered earlier (see p. 14) and are designed to maintain or increase muscle elasticity. They are usually performed within interval or circuit training.

Adaptations related to training methods

Adaptations are actually more directly related to training intensity and duration than they are to training methods. However, the various methods of training offer the best ways of manipulating intensity and duration in order to achieve the desired effect. The table below summarises the relationship between training methods and adaptations.

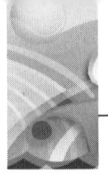

Training stimulus	Adaptations to specific body parts	Anatomical adaptations	Functional adaptations	Training methods that can provide the training stimulus
Aerobic	Cardiovascular	• Increased vascularisation (heart/lungs and muscle tissue) • Increased red blood cell count • Cardiac hypertrophy	• Increased stroke volume • Increased maximal cardiac output • Increased end diastolic volume • Decreased end systolic volume • Bradycardia • Increased VO_2max • Increased efficiency of cardiac and respiratory muscles • Elevation of lactate threshold	Continuous training Long interval training Fartlek training Circuit training Stretching
	Muscular	• Increased vascularisation of localised tissue • Increased production of myoglobin • Increased size and density of mitochondria • Reduction in body fat/increase in lean muscle mass • Increased stores of muscle glycogen	• Increased endurance capacities of localised muscles • Increased efficiency at utilising oxygen	
	Skeletal and connective tissue	• Increased thickness of ligaments and tendons • New stress layers in supporting bones	• Increased elasticity of tendons • Increased strength of ligaments • Increased strength of bones	
	Neuromuscular	• Increased calcium deposits	• Increased capacity for muscle fibre recruitment • Increased capacity for wave summation	
	Other/general	• Increased production of aerobic catalytic enzymes	• Increased metabolic rate • Increased capacity to utilise fat as energy fuel at higher intensity • Increased parasympathethic nervous activity	

Training stimulus	Adaptations to specific body parts	Anatomical adaptations	Functional adaptations	Training methods that can provide the training stimulus
Anaerobic	Cardiovascular	• Increased thickness of ventricular myocardium	• Increased lactic acid tolerance • Increase capacity to tolerate or remove lactic acid	Interval training Speed training Weight/ resistance training Plyometric training SAQ Core stability training
	Muscular	• Increased stores of muscle glycogen • Increased stores of muscular ATP and PC • Hypertrophy of types IIa and IIb fibres	• Increased maximal strength • Increased dynamic strength • Increased power • Increased speed (and acceleration)	
	Skeletal and connective tissue	• Increased thickness of ligaments and tendons • New stress layers in supporting bones	• Increased elasticity of tendons • Increased strength of ligaments • Increased strength of bones	
	Neuromuscular	• Increased calcium deposits	• Increased speed of neural transmission • Increased rate of muscle fibre recruitment • Increased number of muscle fibres recruited	
	Other/general	• Increased production of anaerobic enzymes		

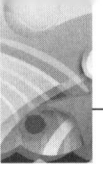

Training stimulus	Adaptations to specific body parts	Anatomical adaptations	Functional adaptations	Training methods that can provide the training stimulus
Threshold	Cardiovascular	• Increased vascularisation (heart/lungs and muscle tissue) • Increased red blood cell count • Cardiac hypertrophy	• Increased stroke volume • Increased maximal cardiac output • Increased end diastolic volume • Decreased end systolic volume • Bradycardia • Increased VO_2max • Increased efficiency of cardiac and respiratory muscles	Fartlek training Circuit training Interval training Speed training Weight/resistance training Core stability training
	Muscular	• Increased vascularisation of localised tissue • Increased production of myoglobin • Increased size and density of mitochondria • Reduction in body fat/increase in lean muscle mass • Increased stores of muscle glycogen	• Increased endurance capacities of localised muscles • Increased efficiency at utilising oxygen	
	Skeletal and connective tissue	• Increased thickness of ligaments and tendons • New stress layers in supporting bones	• Increased elasticity of tendons • Increased strength of ligaments • Increased strength of bones	
	Neuromuscular	• Increased calcium deposits	• Increased speed of neural transmission • Increased capacity to recruit muscle fibres	
	Other/general	• Increased metabolic rate	• Increased VO_2max • Increased lactate tolerance • Increased point of OBLA • Increased speed of recovery	

Tip Make sure that you can say how the different methods of training can be manipulated in order to bring about different and specific structural and ultimately physiological adaptations.

Long-term psychological preparation

Key points

- **Sports psychology** — how this is used in long-term planning.
- **Goal-setting and performance profiling** — uses and benefits.
- **Motivation and attribution theory** — what these are and how they are linked to reviewing/improving performance.
- **Performance development** — using skill development and tactics to improve performance.
- **Group performance and cohesion** — how these can be developed successfully.

We have already discussed how performers use psychological strategies in the short-term preparation phase. Long-term psychological preparation extends these strategies over a longer macrocycle — the actual length of long-term preparation may differ according to the sport and also the cycle of global competition for which an athlete is preparing. The Olympic Games, for example, have a four-year cycle and some athletes will plan their training and competition to peak in four years' time. However, most sports have world championships either annually or in the mid-point between the Olympiads, so many athletes will plan for a one- to two-year macrocycle.

Goal setting and mental training

Mental training is becoming an important element in the long-term preparation phase of elite athletes. Most sports institutes and elite sports squads provide sports psychologists who support athletes in their long-term planning. Key areas that a sport psychologist works on include:

- confidence of the performer
- mental control of the performer
- concentration of the performer

Goal setting is an important part of long-term preparation and will often be linked to the cycle of Olympic Games and world championships. It is best practice to use SMART or SMARTER principles when setting long-term goals.

S pecific	Goals need to be clear, concise and individual.
M easurable	Goals are able to be assessed and reviewed.
A greed	Goals should benefit coaches, team/squad, etc. and be discussed by all.
R ealistic	Goals should be achievable within the timescale given.
T ime-bound	Goals should match the cycle of global sports competitions.
E xciting	Goals should be stimulating and motivating to encourage the performer.
R ecorded	Reviewing and recording progress is an important tool in maintaining commitment and motivating the performer to keep training hard.

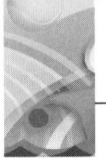

Performance profiling is often linked to goal setting and is normally used as the starting point for the long-term preparation phase. Performance profiling helps athletes by identifying which aspects to concentrate on to achieve optimum performance in sport and how to build these aspects into their training programmes. The process uses a range of feedback techniques in which performances are reviewed, and strengths and weaknesses are identified and analysed.

Most sports in the UK have adopted Long-Term Athlete Development (LTAD) models and these are extensively used in the performance profiling of individual performers. Athletes will use the performance profiling methodology in order to develop a psychological skills training programme.

Long-term psychological training strategies
- Develop imagery techniques
- Use self-talk to help mental control
- Practise mental rehearsal techniques
- Practise progressive relaxation techniques
- Develop strategies that can be used to aid concentration during competition

Motivation and long-term preparation

Success in sport relies on the performer being highly motivated. However, there are many factors, both internal and external, that can affect a performance. In the long-term preparation phase, these factors need to be managed and there needs to be an awareness that motivation levels can change over long periods of time.

There are a number of types of motivation:
- **Intrinsic motivation** — also referred to as primary motivation, this describes internal drives linked to feelings of satisfaction, pleasure and pride. Successful sports performers tend to have high levels of intrinsic motivation.
- **Extrinsic motivation** — also called secondary motivation, this is linked to external rewards or other people. In elite sport, tangible rewards become more important and the extrinsic drive can overtake the intrinsic motivation.
- **Achievement motivation** — this describes the drive to succeed or persist with training or a long-term goal. Closely linked to a performer's personality, elite performers often have high levels of achievement motivation.

Personality and motivation
As defined by Atkinson (1974), there are generally two recognised types of sports personalities: those who 'need to achieve' (Nach) and those who 'need to avoid failure' (Naf). The characteristics of Nach and Naf personalities are shown in the table below.

Nach performers	Naf performers
• Enjoy/choose challenging tasks • Perform better when an audience is present • Perform better when they feel they are being judged • Prefer competitive environments to the practice environment	• Avoid challenge/prefer low risk • Try to avoid shame • Perform less well when they feel they are being judged • Prefer training environments to the competitive environment

Situational factors

The situation in which a performer competes will also influence their motivation levels. Two key situational factors are:

- probability of success versus probability of failure
- incentive value of success versus the incentive value of failure

Other factors influencing motivation include whether performers are:

- **task orientated** — i.e. they focus on performance and process goals
- **ego orientated** — i.e. they are driven by a need to succeed against other people

Attribution theory

Weiner (1974) developed an attribution theory that identifies four main reasons for a result.

	Internal cause	External cause
Stable cause	Ability	Task difficulty
Unstable cause	Effort	Luck

Weiner's attribution theory

When performers suffer a series of defeats or poor performances, they may feel that defeat is inevitable and the result of stable, internal and controllable factors — this is called **learned helplessness**. Attribution retraining can help change attributions to failure and therefore minimise the effects of learned helplessness.

Long-term strategies to develop skills and tactics

- Use visualisation. Creating a mental picture of future success or effective performance also allows athletes to train when they are inured or in rest phases.
- Use mental rehearsal. This allows performers to construct a plan of actions and tactics. It is often used in the final preparation phase but will need to be rehearsed during long-term preparation.
- Use visual awareness training. This means training the eyes and long-term memory to better recognise patterns of play and pick up relevant cues. It is linked to the concept of selective attention.

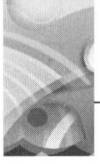

Group cohesion

Many sports require performers to work in groups. Such groups need to work on their cohesion and bonding throughout the long-term preparation phase. The greater the understanding by coaches and performers of the factors that can affect group cohesion, the greater the likelihood of success.

Cohesion of a group has two dimensions:
- **Task cohesion** — working together to achieve agreed common goals and tasks.
- **Social cohesion** — the friendship of the group; groups work well together when the individual members enjoy each other's company.

The development of sports groups normally goes through four stages:
1 **Forming** — the group is created/selected.
2 **Storming** — roles are identified and tasks allocated.
3 **Norming** — cohesion develops, rules and standards are agreed.
4 **Performing** — the group matures and works effectively.

> **Strategies for enhancing group cohesion**
> To enhance environmental factors:
> - Use training camps.
> - All players should be given equal importance and praise.
>
> To enhance personal factors:
> - All members should share ownership of the group.
> - Break up any cliques or subgroups within the team.
>
> To enhance leadership factors:
> - Use a mixture of leadership styles.
> - Be aware of each player's needs.
>
> To enhance team factors:
> - Use team goals and planning.
> - All members of the team should have a clear role.

Long-term technical preparation

Key points

- **Mechanical aspects of long-term preparation** — what these are and how they can be used to refine technique and develop perfect models.
- **Technology and feedback** — how these are used in long-term sports preparation.
- **Ergogenic aids** — how these are used over the long term in sport.

Long-term preparation take place well before competition. The aim is to adapt fitness, technique and skills so that the performer works more efficiently and ultimately improves their performance. Though in the past the main emphasis has been on physiological training and adaptation, in modern sport elite athletes need to work on all aspects — physiological, psychological and mechanical. We have already discussed the long-term preparation in physiological and psychological areas. This section focuses on the mechanical area of sports preparation.

Mechanical aspects of long-term preparation

Mechanical preparation involves a wide range of areas, including:
- using biomechanics to review and improve the movements of sporting action
- designing clothing and equipment to give performance a competitive edge
- using video and computer software to identify weaknesses in technique

The main aim of long-term mechanical preparation is to refine the techniques of performers and teams. By producing a greater efficiency of movement, mechanical preparation can maximise the impact of physical effort.

The basic method of technical support is the review of performance in order to identify strengths and weaknesses or areas for improvement. Using this analysis, adjustments can be suggested that will rectify the weaknesses. The performer will try these in practice, and then in competition, and then the whole process will start again.

Refining technique and developing perfect models

Good technique in sport is a result of a well-timed and coordinated sequence of movements. Developing correct technique as part of the long-term preparation phase is beneficial to performers as it:
- improves performance
- makes better use of energy and power
- reduces the risk of injury

Techniques in all sports are constantly changing, and performers and coaches need to keep up to date with technique development in their sport. This can be done by attending coaching conferences, analysing the performance of other performers and keeping up to date with sport-specific publications.

Improvements in a performer's technique can be developed through the application of basic mechanical principles:
- ensuring that the performer is applying forces in the correct direction
- ensuring that the posture of the performer is in the most effective form
- identifying possible overuse injuries by reviewing the forces and motion of the performer's actions

Key areas that the performer may focus on in the long-term preparation phase could include developing technique in terms of:
- coordination
- positional awareness
- peripheral vision training/sports vision training
- running technique
- grip (racket sports)
- posture
- repetitive actions, such as kicking or throwing

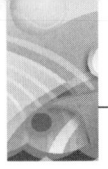

Most performers and their coaches work towards a **perfect model** — the recognised way of executing a particular skill or action. Increasingly, this model may well be computer-generated. Video and computer software is also used extensively to help performers review their performance. Commercial packages, such as Dartfish and Prozone, are able to give detailed feedback and analysis on a range of sports performances.

Use of ergogenic aids in long-term preparation

Ergogenic aids are any external influence that can be used to improve performance. We have previously discussed the use of ergogenic aids in the short-term preparation phase. Some of those strategies can also be used in the long-term phase.

Ergogenic aids used in the long-term phase can enhance physiological, psychological, nutritional and chemical adaptations. Performers are always striving to find the competitive edge and this why many use ergogenic aids in their long-term preparation. Chemical ergogenic aids, such as food supplements, are used to enable performers to train for longer and at higher intensity.

Examples of ergogenic aids used in long-term preparation include:
- **Force plates** — these are used to measure and give feedback on fitness components such as power and muscular endurance.
- **Pedometers** — by measuring steps per minute, known as pedometry, a performer can obtain feedback on the distances covered during practice or competition. Pedometers can also be used to help calculate energy expenditure.
- **Heart-rate monitors** — heart-rate monitoring allows athletes to work within training zones that are matched to heart-rate levels.
- **GPS devices** — GPS technology is used in endurance sport to give feedback on distance covered, maximum and average speed.

Clothing and equipment design in sport

What players wear and use can have a huge impact on performance. These items are designed and developed over the long term to give performers the competitive edge. Key areas include:
- **Aero and fluid dynamics** — clothing is designed that will enable the performer to move more quickly and efficiently through the air or water.
- **Thermoregulation** — garments are designed that can either maintain heat, for example in a sprinter's lower legs, or cool down a performer's temperature, for example for endurance cycling or running.
- **Weight** — lighter equipment, such as rackets and cycles, are designed so that performers need to use less energy moving around unwanted weight.
- **Friction** — footwear is designed that either produces more grip, for example in football or golf, or reduces friction, for example in sprinting, thereby creating more efficient movement.
- **Recovery** — compression clothing is designed to encourage circulation and so speed up recovery rates.
- **Power** — a recent innovation, ionized clothing, claims to increase power and endurance.

Managing elite performance

Centres of excellence

Key points

- **Historical development** — how elite sports support emerged.
- **Global case studies** — an overview of four different systems of support for elite sports (East Germany, USA, Australia and UK).
- **Elite athletes** — what they need in order to maintain their high standards.
- **The academy system of support** — its benefits for elite sports.

In the twenty-first century, elite performers and teams spend vast amounts of time and resources preparing for global competitions. This section investigates how elite athletes are supported around the world. It considers the history of support for elite sports, identifying the key stages of development and discussing the different types of support that different countries use. It also discusses the benefits and issues relating to the use of sports institutes and academies.

History and development of elite sports support

Early history

The concept of sporting excellence emerged in the UK with the rise of professional sportsmen during the seventeenth and early eighteenth centuries. Early professionals were mainly paid retainers, employed by the upper classes to train and prepare for sports competitions.

The public schools of the nineteenth century

By the late nineteenth century, the best performers were drawn exclusively from the middle and upper classes, who had been nurtured through the public schools system with its philosophy of 'Muscular Christianity' and the games ethic. Fee-paying boarding schools provided pupils with both the time and facilities to practise and compete in a range of sports. The influence of these schools, as discussed in Unit 1, was huge and most of the sports played by their pupils became the standard sports in global competitions, such as the newly established Olympics Games that arrived in 1896. Many public schools began to employ professional players, whose role was to coach and provide the pupils with skilful opponents. This was the first attempt in the UK at systematic sports preparation.

The Oxbridge universities

When boys left public school, many would then continue their studies at the universities of Oxford and Cambridge. They took the development of sport to the next level, helping to establish the first form of standardised rules and establishing competitive sport. Oxbridge athletes figured largely in the formation of rules, national associations and international and domestic amateur sports teams.

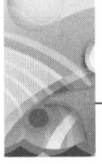

The expanding British empire

Rational sport quickly spread throughout the British empire. Many countries adopted the sports that had been developed in the UK and soon international fixtures began to develop. It was quickly recognised that sport offered an opportunity to test oneself against athletes from other nations.

The modern Olympic Games

Baron de Coubertin's vision of an international sports festival that would allow the best performers from around the globe to meet and compete every 4 years was realised in 1896 when the Athens Games became the first of the modern Olympics. Almost immediately, performers and their nations began taking preparation seriously in order to improve their chances of wining medals.

The US college athletes — the first elite

The US team 'won' the first games in 1896. The US was already involved in systematic training, drawing the majority of its Olympic team from the collegiate systems. US universities had already begun supporting elite athletes, offering a balance of study and training time and facilities.

The Cold War and superpower rivalry

The re alignment of states in Eastern Europe following the Second World War created the so-called Eastern Bloc. These communist nations recognised that success in global sport had an important role in promoting both internal morale and external pride. Every aspect of sporting excellence, from selection to training and diet, was coordinated by the central government.

Twenty-first century globalisation

The globalisation of sport and the continued development of emergent cultures has meant that virtually all countries now have a planned elite sports programme. Most nations competing in global games have developed central training bases for their top athletes, usually a national institute of sport, and have also developed support mechanisms to help fund and develop the performance of their elite sports squads.

The academy model

One of the constant features of elite sports systems is the use of specialist sports academies or institutes to prepare elite athletes. First developed in East Germany in the 1960s, these centres offer elite training facilities and the support network (e.g. sports science, medical, coaching services) that have now become essential elements of elite sports preparation. In some cases these are residential centres where athletes live and train for long periods.

Elite sport in different cultures

East Germany

East Germany (which is no longer a separate country) was one of the first nations to develop a state-run elite sports system, including screening of potential talent at primary school, plus the creation of sports schools and specialist sports institutes. East Germany's approach to the achievement of excellence during its brief 41-year history shaped programmes across the world for the next century. Despite having a population of only 16 million, East Germany achieved a high degree of global sports success.

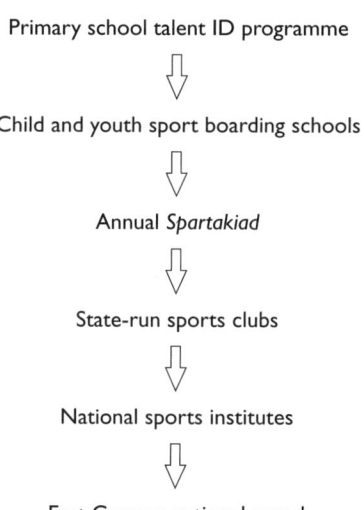

Primary school talent ID programme

Child and youth sport boarding schools

Annual *Spartakiad*

State-run sports clubs

National sports institutes

East German national squad

The East German elite sports pathway

Primary school talent ID programme
Full-time specialist PE teachers, coaches and medical staff would screen all pupils for potential sporting talent.

Child and youth sports boarding school
Those who showed potential in one of the state's list of programme sports would be sent to one of the country's 25 child and youth sport schools. Here, young people trained for over 50 hours a week in their specific sports, with full-time coaches.

Annual Spartakiads
Spartakiads or mini-Olympics were held in order to replicate the pressures of global sports competition.

State-run sports clubs
All sport schools were linked to state-run sports clubs. Often these would be associated with a particular trade union. They allowed sportsmen and women to train and perform full-time without jeopardising their Olympic amateur status.

National sports institutes
A series of national sports institutes had state-of-the-art facilities for athletes to train and be monitored in. They were used for the final stage of preparation in the run-up to the Olympic Games and other major championships.

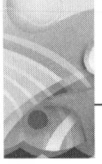

Australia

The Australian Institute of Sport (AIS) has led the development of elite sport in Australia for over 25 years. The AIS was created following Australia's disappointing performance at the 1976 Olympics in Montreal, in which they won just one silver medal and four bronze medals. The federal government conducted a review of the nation's elite sport system, and concluded that Australia needed a centre of excellence that would prepare athletes for international competition. The AIS's role in developing sports excellence can be judged by the fact that at the 1992 Barcelona Olympics, Australia won 27 medals, including seven golds.

Modified sports programmes

⇩

Talent ID programmes

⇩

Sports clubs and regional zones

⇩

State-level sport

⇩

National sports institutes
AIS and state institutes

⇩

Australian national squad
or
Full-time professional sport

The Australian elite sports pathway

Modified sports programmes

Each Australian sport has developed a junior version that develops the basic skills required in the sport. Examples include Netta netball and Auskick football.

Talent ID programmes

The Australian Sports Commission manages a national talent identification and development programme that aims to identify potential athletes who can be fast tracked into sport-specific programmes at regional and state level.

Sports clubs and regional zones

Performers then transfer into club sport, which is tiered in terms of ability in most local areas. Talented performers will then get the chance to represent their region.

State-level sport

Most sports in Australia have a state-level team. These play in annual 'state of origin' competitions.

National sports institutes — AIS and state institutes

State institutes are non-residential and provide a central location for management, coaches, athlete support and sports science and medical support. The AIS offers scholarships every year to almost 600 athletes in 32 separate programmes covering 25 sports, and employs around 75 full-time coaches in a range of sports. The AIS provides Australian athletes with world-class training facilities, high-performance coaching, state-of-the-art equipment, and a world-class sports medicine and sports science facility.

USA

The development of elite sport in the USA is focused exclusively on the school and college system — this is completely different from the club-based approach in most European countries. High school and college sport in the USA is a mirror of the professional sports system. Most high schools have lavish facilities for both players and spectators. Students move first from high school onto scholarship programmes for various sports at college level. Then, if they are good enough, they enter the **annual draft**. Although this is the dream of all aspiring school athletes, it must be noted that this is an elitist and competitive selection process, with fewer than 4% of high school first team players progressing to the draft stage of recruitment.

Little League sport

⇩

High school sports programmes

⇩

Athletic scholarships at HE colleges

⇩

Annual draft

⇩

Full-time professional sport

The US elite sports pathway

Little League sport

Modified versions of US sports for children are known as Little Leagues. These are highly competitive games that mirror their adult versions in terms of organisation and competition structure.

High school sports programmes

Inter-school sport reaches its greatest intensity in grades 11 and 12 (ages 16–18), when students represent their school first team in various sports. Most games take place on a Friday night, attracting a large community following.

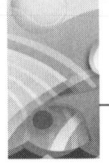

Athletic scholarships at HE colleges

Talented performers are offered athletic scholarships to cover academic costs and allow them to train and compete while gaining an education. Many sports are high profile and run as professional/commercial enterprises.

Annual draft

Every college game is recorded and analysed by a national office, which then scores and ranks every college player across the states, identifying the best athletes to go forward into the draft. For the major professional sports, this is the only route into the professional ranks. The weakest professional team from the previous season gets the first pick of the best college athletes.

UK

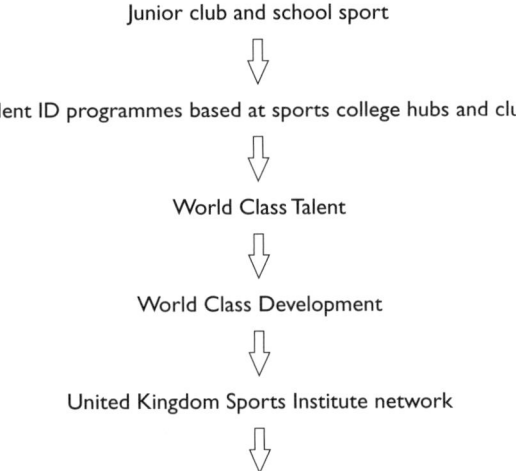

Junior club and school sport

⇩

Talent ID programmes based at sports college hubs and clubs

⇩

World Class Talent

⇩

World Class Development

⇩

United Kingdom Sports Institute network

⇩

World Class Podium

The UK elite sports pathway

World Class Talent/Development/Podium

The World Class Pathway funds the performance and subsistence costs of UK elite athletes. The funding comes from the Sports Lottery fund via the athlete's home sports council. The programme aims to invest world-class funds to achieve consistent success in top-level international competitions, such as the Olympic, Paralympic and World Deaf Games.

Teams and individuals on the World Class programme must pass agreed selection criteria before they are nominated by their respective governing bodies. The programme has three stages, with the amount of support and funding available increasing as athletes move towards the World Class Podium level. However, all athletes on the programme have access to the network centres (see below).

The funding of elite athletes in the UK is made up of two parts:
- **Programme funding** — this is given to sports governing bodies to cover support

services to athletes, such as coaching and medical staff, warm-weather training and sports science.
- **Athlete personal awards** — this is given to individual performers to help support their living costs and sporting costs (the average grant is £10,000–12,000).

Currently, the World Class Performance programme supports 24 sports and 730 athletes, with a budget of around £20 million a year. This funding relies wholly on the public's purchase of tickets for the Wednesday and Saturday night National Lottery draws. Much of the early support and talent identification is offered through the school sports partnership programme and in particular through schools with specialist status for sport.

United Kingdom Sports Institute (UKSI) network

The UKSI network of elite training and research centres assists governing bodies and their top performers in preparing for international and global championships. These centres provide state-of-the art facilities, as well as support from sports scientists, medical professionals, coaches and support personnel.

Other elite sports initiatives include:
- **National governing bodies** — many continue to develop their excellence and talent identification programmes.
- **Elite Coach education programme** — elite coaches are offered a range of training programmes and resources to aid in their coaching.
- **UK Centre for Coaching Excellence** — to be based at Leeds Carnegie University, this will offer a coaching faculty that will pass on expertise to coaches.
- **Performance lifestyle (formerly ACE UK)** — a national programme that aims to enhance an athlete's personal development and sporting performance by offering services such as career advice, educational support, personal finance training, media and presentation skills training.

Support roles and finance

The increasing standard of elite sports competition makes it extremely difficult for athletes to compete for medals. In the twenty-first century, virtually all athletes in all sports now have to train full time.

In the past, countries such as the USA and the Soviet Union funded athletes indirectly through the armed forces or student grants. Increasingly, over the past few decades, more and more countries are now funding their athletes directly in order to allow them to train on a full-time basis.

The funding of elite athletes differs around the world. There are four main methods of financially supporting elite performers:
- funding directly from the state
- funding from charities and private institutions, such as lotteries, pools, sports institutes
- sponsorship, such as Nike Running Camps
- salaried sports, including traditional professional sports such as soccer and rugby league

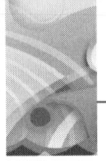

Elite performers will use this personal funding to cover the costs of travelling to training and competition, entry fees, training and medical support, as well as taking a basic salary.

State funding — the debate

There are many who argue against direct state funding for elite performers. It can be claimed that such money might be better spent at the base of the participation pyramid, where it could have an impact on many more individuals. Research suggests that on average it costs several millions pounds to support one athlete who wins an Olympic medal. This does not seem to be an efficient system. The suggested impact of successful athletes becoming role models and so inspiring the next generation to take up sport is also based more on myth than fact. There is no point in being inspired to take up a sport such as rowing or sailing if there is no provision for these sports in your local area.

State funding also makes sport a political tool, and there may be pressure on athletes to compete and travel to particular countries and competitions to suit their government's agenda. Finally, the USA — the most successful nation in Olympic history — does not publicly fund any of its Olympic teams or individual athletes.

Recent research by PricewaterhouseCoopers (June 2008) found a direct link between state funding and the number of medals a nation wins. This was particularly important to nations with small populations, such as East Germany and Australia, which have a smaller pool of talent from which to select. This Australian research suggested that each gold medal cost on average US$37 million worth of funding.

Private sector academies

There are an increasing number of private companies and professional sports clubs that are establishing sports academies. These tend to charge participants a fee for the services provided — and in return they supply top-class facilities and high-level coaching, often from former top-class performers. Most of these private sector academies offer short, intensive courses that often coincide with school holidays, rather than full-time residential support, as in the case of the publicly funded sports institutes.

Training for the Olympic Games

Training camps are used by international sports teams in the weeks and months before major competitions. They are extensively used by teams preparing for Olympic, Paralympic and Commonwealth Games. In the UK, the British Olympic Association differentiates between two sorts of camp when supporting Team GB in its preparation for the Olympic and Paralympic Games.

Holding camps:

- are single-base camps used in the weeks immediately prior to the start of the games
- help athletes to acclimatise to the competition conditions by matching the climate, altitude and time zone of the host city
- help athletes to improve focus and maximise their performance at the games

Preparation camps:
- use the same facilities as the holding camp but are used up to a year before the event
- enable athletes, coaches and support staff to familiarise themselves with the location
- allow the team to have a 'dry run' of procedures and transfer arrangements

Needs of elite athletes
Elite athletes require access to exclusive training facilities in the 2–3 weeks prior to a major event. These facilities need to be of a high standard. The location needs to have similar climatic conditions and the same time zone as the competition venue. Support facilities need to include access to a hospital with an Accident and Emergency department with advanced scanner technology. The camp also needs to be within half a day's direct flight from the host city in order to avoid travel fatigue.

Technical support

Key points
- **The role of technology in training analysis** — how elite athletes use technology to give feedback on performance.
- **Sports science support** — how technology and sports science can be used for the enhancement and evaluation of sporting performance.
- **The support of national agencies** — how national agencies support the preparation of elite athletes.

In order to reach their optimum performance level, modern sports performers require support from a range of sports science disciplines. In most sports these include:
- physiology
- biomechanics
- nutrition
- sports psychology

Much of this support is now provided by sports academies and institutes, where athletes can train and receive detailed feedback that enables them and their coaches to modify and optimise their training programmes. The process of using technical feedback to analyse and review a performer's development is known as **performance analysis**.

An example of performance analysis is the notational analysis system used in professional sports to study a team's strategy and tactics. Notational analysis focuses on gross movements or movement patterns within a team. For example, in football, notational analysis could provide feedback on:
- match indicators — shots on target, shots off target, number of corners, crosses, fouls committed

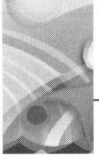

- technical indicators — number of passes, dribbles, lost control, tackles won, tackles lost
- tactical indicators — time in possession, passing distribution, possession linked to pitch position

Role of technology in training analysis

With so much at stake, elite performers are always searching for a competitive edge, which will allow them to perform slightly better than their opponents. It is in finding this edge that technology has played an increasingly important role in elite sport.

Sports technology can be used to improve performance in two main ways:
(1) helping the performer to perfect technique through the use of analysis
(2) refining the playing kit and equipment used to give the performer a competitive edge

Technological advances have had so much influence in some sports that the rules have had to be changed. There is some debate whether technology in sport fits with concept of fair play and the spirit of sport. If it is available only to an exclusive group of athletes (those who can afford to access it), technology could be seen as cheating. Only if athletes have equal access to the technology will their success be solely dependent on the ability and skill of the individual athlete.

Technology appears to have the greatest impact on sports that involve gross motor skills and movements such as sprinting. It would appear that technology has less impact than in sports where more techniques and fine skills are required.

Sports manufacturers such as Nike and Speedo spend millions of dollars each year on research to develop footwear and swimsuits that could help shave vital milliseconds off world records. However, research and analysis of results suggest that, in many of these sports, the impact has been minimal.

Sports science and support of elite athletes

The influence of sports science is now found in every aspect of a performer's training, preparation and performance analysis. Elite performers have their training schedule prepared by sports science experts, to ensure they are doing the right kinds of training to match the specific demands of their sport and position, so that they will be in a peak physical and mental state for their competitions.

Their diet and fluid intake is measured, monitored and adjusted by sports scientists. Their clothing and equipment has been designed by sports scientists to ensure they can perform at their optimum level.

Once athletes have completed their performance, statisticians, video reviewers and coaches analyse their performance, giving detailed feedback and advice about what went right and wrong, and how they can improve future performance.

The main support roles of sports scientists, and how they affect training and performance, are listed below.

- **Exercise physiologists** — help optimise training objectives and ensure that the performers follow prescribed training that is specific to the demands of their sport and position.
- **Sports psychologists** — help athletes to prepare mentally for competition. This may involve helping performers to deal with feelings of arousal.
- **Nutrionists** — assist athletes in choosing the right food and fluids in the right amounts, and in taking these at the right time to meet the demands of training and competition.
- **Biomechanists** — help athletes to develop better and more efficient techniques so ensuring a higher level of performance and also reducing the risk of injury.
- **Sports vision specialists** — work on assessment and enhancement of sports performers' use of vision. They develop training programmes that improve visual acuity, hand–eye coordination, peripheral vision, perception and reaction time.
- **Sports podiatrists** — analyse how performers feet strike the ground, highlighting any mechanical problems that could lead to injury. This information is used to refine the performers' technique, and possibly to add orthotic aids to the performers' footwear.

Role of national agencies

At the turn of the twenty-first century, the provision of high-quality coaching, science and medical support services has become essential in the preparation of elite sports performers.

The former Eastern Bloc countries were the first nations to fully develop support programmes for their elite athletes, but by the mid-1990s most governments had developed their own elite sports programmes and/or national training centres. Reasons for this include the fact that sport plays an increasingly important role in most modern global societies. The increasing level of media attention and the national honour and international prestige that global success brings are also contributory factors.

The sports science support outlined above is normally provided and funded via national sports agencies within a country. There are two main models in global sport:
(1) **the centralised model** — elite sports are supported via the state, which appoints a central body to oversee the management of the country's elite sports programme. Examples include the Australian and French elite sports systems.
(2) **the decentralised model** — no single agency takes control, but there is a developed system of supporting elite sport through higher education institutions. Examples include the USA scholarship system

Most elite sport programmes target performers at a young age. Any young performer who shows above-average sporting ability is generally encouraged to attend regular coaching and development sessions at regional centres of sports excellence. The objective of these satellite elite training centres is to create an environment that nurtures the performance of the young athletes. Support is given to aid the athletes

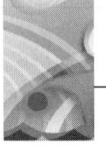

with both physical and psychological development, as well as helping them to cope with the demands of global sports competitions.

Many of these training centres are classified as academies and often represent the first step towards a career in elite sport. Academies usually focus on young people aged 14–18 and allow performers to combine elite sports training with academic education. Research suggests that the average age of Olympic champions is decreasing. Currently the average age for most sports is the early twenties.

Elite training centres and academies offer practice and training conditions that are as close as possible to the competitive environment. Their use is often exclusive to the elite teams and athletes, so that there are no distractions or issues over access.

Questions & Answers

This section contains questions similar in style to those you can expect to see in the Unit 3 examination. The limited number of example questions means that it is impossible to cover all the topics and all the question styles, but they should give you a flavour of what to expect. The responses shown are real students' answers to the questions.

There are several ways of using this section:

- Hide the answers and try the questions yourself. It needn't be a memory test — use your notes to see whether you can make all the points you need to. Remember, you need to include a sufficient number of points to match the mark allocation for the question.
- Check your answers against the candidates' responses and make an estimate of the likely standard of your response to each question.
- Check your answers against the examiner's comments to see if you can appreciate where you might have lost marks.
- Check your answers against the terms used in the question — did you *explain* or *discuss* when you were asked to, or did you merely *describe*?

Examiner's comments

All candidate responses are followed by examiner's comments. These are preceded by the icon ℮ and indicate where credit is due. In the weaker answers, they also point out areas for improvement, specific problems and common errors, such as lack of clarity, weak or non-existent development, irrelevance, misinterpretation of the question and mistaken meanings of terms.

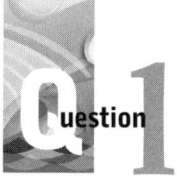

Warming up

Identify the stages to a warm-up and state the type of activity that would be done in each stage. (6 marks)

■ ■ ■

✍ Any of the following marking points would receive 1 mark:
- Initial preparation/heart rate elevation/pulse raiser
- e.g. gross motor skill such as jogging
- Injury prevention
- e.g. mobility exercises such as stretching
- Skills practice
- e.g. skills in isolation/lower intensity
- Sports specific
- e.g. high tempo skills/as in a game

■ ■ ■

Candidates' answers to Question 1

Candidate A

When warming up you should first go for a run, this will warm your muscles and your body up. Next you should stretch out your muscles, this will increase your flexibility. After that you should practise some of the skills that you will use. This will help to improve your concentration and your timing. All of this shows how a warm-up can improve your performance.

✍ Everything that the candidate has written is accurate with regards to warming up. However, much of it was not required by the question and so is a waste of time. The candidate also fails to identify by name any of the stages and so loses those marks. 3 marks have been scored for listing the three types of activities performed.

Candidate B

There are three stages of a warm-up, which are initial preparation, injury prevention and skills practice. You would do different activities within each stage. For a footballer you would do some jogging in the first stage, stretch your quadriceps and hamstring in the second stage and do some passing or some heading in the third stage.

✍ An excellent answer and one that illustrates that if you answer the question you do not always have to write large amounts of content. This candidate scores 3 marks in the first sentence and then goes on to accurately, and with the help of an applied example of football, state the activities would be completed in each stage. The answer scores 6 out of 6.

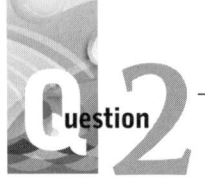

Question 2

Home advantage

Explain the positive and negative effects on performance of competing in front of a home crowd. (3 marks)

■ ■ ■

A maximum of 2 marks is available for explaining positive effects, and a maximum of 2 marks for negative effects. A total of 3 marks can therefore be achieved from the content points below.

Positive:
- The away team may be put off by a hostile home crowd
- The away team may play more aggressively and give away more fouls
- The home team receives support/encouragement from the home crowd
- The home team's knowledge of the surroundings/equipment/court/pitch will have a positive influence on performance

Negative:
- An increased feeling of pressure to do well may lead to a drop in the home team's performance
- An increase in arousal may lead to the home team becoming over aroused and dropping performance level/inverted U theory/catastrophe theory
- The home team may lose the support of the home crowd if mistakes are made/evaluation apprehension/loss of self-confidence

■ ■ ■

Candidates' answers to Question 2

Candidate A

Positive
The home crowd will give lots of support to the players, which will make them more confident and perform to a higher level.

Playing at home also means that the players will be used to the pitch dimensions and therefore feel more confident and play better.

Negative
Playing in front of a home crowd can put the players under more pressure to perform well — this could affect their stress and anxiety levels.

If the performance is not very good then the crowd may start to get at the players and this may affect their confidence levels.

This answer scores the maximum 3 marks. The candidate makes good points and clearly states both positive and negative effects. It is good practice to use headings from the question to help structure your answer and ensure that both you and the examiner see that you are answering the question.

Candidate B

Playing at home can have both positive and negative effects on the performance of a team or individual. The home supporters can both help the team in terms of giving their support but their presence may cause a drop in performance. The support from the home crowd will give the home players a lot of confidence and make them feel good about themselves. This will normally have a positive effect on performance. However, the need to perform well in front of the home crowd can lead to a rise in anxiety and this may mean some players underperform and will lose confidence and this will be a negative effect.

This answer includes one positive and one negative effect and therefore scores 2 marks. Candidate B has wasted valuable effort in repeating the question.

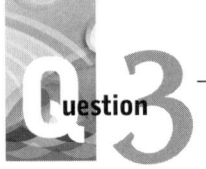

Use of ergogenic aids

Explain why athletes are increasingly using ergogenic aids in their short-term preparation for optimum sports performance. (4 marks)

■ ■ ■

Any four from the following marking points:
- Margins are narrow in global sports/hundredths of a second can determine who wins. Ergogenic aids can give performers a competitive edge
- Most elite athletes now follow similar training programmes/diets. Many are looking to try something new
- Elite athletes now have access to teams of sports scientists who are developing ergogenic aids
- Ergogenic aids are a reflection of the more technical/scientific approach to sport
- Most ergogenic aids remain legal, e.g. use of supplements
- The demands of modern sport mean that athletes have to recover more quickly/play more matches. Ergogenic aids can help recovery
- Increased funding of sport/commercialisation of sport means that more money is available to develop ergogenic aids

■ ■ ■

Candidates' answers to Question 3

Candidate A

There are four main types of ergogenic aids used in elite sport.

Mechanical ergogenic aids. These involve using technology such as a heart-rate monitor to identify training thresholds and allow a performer to train at a specific level to better develop their fitness for their sport.

Chemical ergogenic aids. These are supplements or drugs that help athletes to train harder or recover more quickly — modern sport requires players to play a lot more games so this is very important.

Physiological ergogenic aids. These include using things like acupuncture and massage to help athletes prepare for competition.

Psychological ergogenic aids. Using imagery, music and hypnosis can help athletes to mentally prepare for competition.

This candidate, though making valid points, is not answering the question. The answer describes the types of ergogenic aids an athlete can use but does not, in the main, explain *why* athletes may have increased their use of ergogenic aids. A 'benefit of the doubt' (BOD) mark would be awarded for the point about the increasing demands of modern sport. This answer would therefore score 1 mark only.

Remember, it is vital to read the question carefully. If needed, use a highlighter pen to pick out the exam command word (in this case *explain*) and any other key points that you need to cover in your exam answer.

Candidate B

In modern sport, the margins between winning and losing are very narrow — elite athletes are always seeking the extra edge that will make them the winner. This is why many now take and use a range of ergogenic aids. The best examples include supplements, such as creatine, which athletes use to make sure their PC energy stores are at their highest.

Most elite athletes are also based at sports institutes where they will have access to a wide range of ergogenic aids — it is almost expected now that elite athletes need to use ergogenic aids if they want to be successful. There is also a lot more money available to elite athletes — lottery funding and sponsorship means that they have more money to spend on ergogenic aids.

This candidate makes a good attempt at answering the question and includes three relevant points. The answer therefore scores 3 marks. Remember to write enough points to match the marks available for the question.

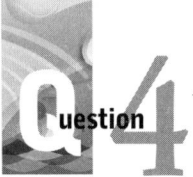

Effects of altitude

Identify and explain the initial effects of altitude upon aerobic performance.

(6 marks)

■ ■ ■

🖉 A maximum of 3 marks are available for identifying the effects, and 3 marks available for explanation. Each of the following marking points would score 1 mark:

Identification of effects:
- Increased heart rate
- Reduced VO_2max
- Lower anaerobic threshold for a given exercise output (i.e. running speed)
- Reduced performance/harder to exercise at the same level

Explanation of effects:
- Higher altitude has a lower air pressure. Although O_2 is of a similar percentage within a given quantity of air, the volume of air is expanded so the O_2 is spread over a larger area
- Consequently O_2 exerts a lower partial pressure at altitude
- Produces a lower pressure gradient
- Less O_2 enters the body/lower level of haemoglobin saturation
- Less O_2 means reaching anaerobic levels sooner

■ ■ ■

Candidates' answers to Question 4

Candidate A

When training at altitude an aerobic athlete would find it much harder because there is less oxygen in the air.

This would mean that they could not get enough oxygen into their bodies to be able to perform as well as at sea level.

Consequently they would get tired quicker and have to slow down or stop, giving them a worse performance.

🖉 The candidate understood that there were two parts to the question and has attempted to answer both parts (although in reverse order). However, the answer lacks sufficient accuracy and detail to score the available 6 marks.

To say 'there is less oxygen in the air' is a common error and does not receive a mark. Air pressure is lower at altitude and so the volume of air is spread over a greater area giving a lower density of air. However there is still approximately 19% of O_2 for any given unit of air, as there is at sea level.

The candidate makes two scoring points: the fact that less oxygen can enter the body and the fact that performance is made worse. So in total the candidate only scored 2 of the available 6 marks, mainly due to an answer that was too brief, was a little repetitive and lacked sufficient accuracy.

Candidate B

The initial effect of altitude on performance would be that performance is not as good as when at sea level. The athlete would have a higher heart rate because there is less oxygen entering the bloodstream and so the heart has to work faster to circulate more oxygen. Because they have a higher heart rate they would reach their maximum heart rate sooner. All of this is down to the lower pp of oxygen at altitude.

Most of what this candidate has written is accurate and so would score marks. The answer is relatively concise and there is no repetition. However, the candidate has jumped about a little with regards to the two things required by the question and so has not provided enough content to score the full allocation of marks available. If you look back at the available marking points you will see that this answer would score 4 marks.

Plyometrics

Using a named plyometric exercise, explain the concepts behind this type of training. (4 marks)

■ ■ ■

Each of the following marking points would score 1 mark:
- Example of a plyometric exercise, such as bounding
- The force generated by landing forcibly stretches the quadriceps muscle
- This is an eccentric contraction
- If the quadriceps immediately perform a concentric contraction/second jump...
- ...the stretch reflex action produces a greater force than normal
- Good training for generating power/coordination

■ ■ ■

Candidates' answers to Question 5

Candidate A

Plyometrics involves a muscle performing an eccentric contraction by acting as a brake. The muscle then contracts concentrically and because of the first contraction it is able to generate more force.

This is an excellent description of the principle of plyometrics with good and accurate use of technical language. The candidate fails to identify an exercise and so loses 1 mark, and as a consequence is unable to relate the answer to the exercise (which would have gained another mark). The answer therefore scores 2 out of 4 marks, but with just a little more detail and a named exercise could have scored the full 4 marks.

Candidate B

Plyometrics are good for developing power but they should not be used too often as they can cause DOMS.

Examples of plyometric exercises are clap press-ups, bounding, depth box jumps, throwing and catching a medicine ball.

Plyometrics is a good method of training because it can be made quite sport specific.

Once again, this answer contains accurate information regarding plyometrics, but a lot of it is irrelevant to the question. Potential negative effects are not required, nor are additional examples and benefits. More attention needs to be given to explaining the concept. In total, 2 out of 4 marks are scored.

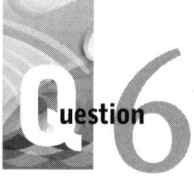

Interval training

Athletes often use interval training as a training method to enhance performance. Identify the characteristics of interval training, explaining why it is such a popular method.
(4 marks)

■ ■ ■

The marking points are as follows:
- Training based on a work:rest (W:R) ratio
- Repeated
- Very adaptable/flexible
- Different fitness benefits can be obtained
- Quick/avoids boredom
- Can be very sport specific

■ ■ ■

Candidates' answers to Question 6

Candidate A

Interval training is training with gaps or breaks in it.

It is used by sprinters and other anaerobic type athletes.

It develops power and speed.

The best thing about this answer is that the candidate sets out the three points that they wanted to make quite clearly. However, the answer fails to score any marks. The definition is too vague — 'with gaps or breaks in it' could be referring to a day, two days or even weeks. Interval training can be used by sprinters and it can be manipulated to develop power or speed, however it is not exclusive to this. Consequently 0 marks are scored.

Candidate B

Interval training is exercise that has regular or set breaks between sets, you work for a period of time and then rest. The sets are repeated several times. It can be used by a lot of different types of athletes because you can adapt it to suit whatever you are doing. And so you can get a variety of different fitness benefits.

An excellent answer that is worth the maximum marks. Each sentence appears on the list of markable points and so receives 1 mark.

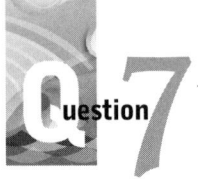

Question 7

Circuit training

Describe the main concepts of circuit training and identify the benefits associated with it. (4 marks)

■ ■ ■

✐ Each of the following marking points would be awarded 1 mark:
- Athletes perform different exercises at different stations
- Working different body parts/performing different skills
- Can be quick
- Not boring
- Rapid results
- Enables body parts/systems/skills to be overloaded
- Provides multiple benefits/adaptable

■ ■ ■

Candidates' answers to Question 7

Candidate A

Circuit training involves you working at different stations in order or sequence. You perform different exercises at each station. Because of this you can get a lot of different fitness benefits in one exercise period. You can perform exercises for speed at one station, flexibility at the next, endurance at the next and maximal strength at the next.

✐ There is a promising start to this answer with a very good definition of circuit training to score 1 mark. However, the candidate then proceeds to demonstrate that they are actually confused by the concept of this method of training. You can use circuit training to achieve a variety of different components of fitness but not in the same circuit. You need to design a circuit for a specific component.

Candidate B

Circuit training is when you move from exercise station to station and perform different exercises.

It is popular because it can be done quickly and adapted to suit whatever sport you play.

You can also get a full body work-out by alternating the exercises at each station between different body parts.

This can make it enjoyable and fun

✐ As you can see this is an excellent answer that had sufficient accurate information to score 5 marks. Each sentence could score a mark, but of course the candidate can only receive the maximum 4 marks that were available.

Attribution theory

Discuss how a coach could use their knowledge of attribution theory to increase the confidence of a sports performer as part of their long-term preparation.

(4 marks)

■ ■ ■

Each of the following marking points would score 1 mark:

- Attribute good play to internal factors, e.g. effort and skill, which are controllable by the performer
- Attribute losing to unstable factors/point out that things could be different next time
- Tell the player they will win because they are good enough/they have trained well and are prepared
- Tell the player that not training/trying hard enough will result in a poor performance and losses
- Attribute poor performance to external factors
- Undertake attribution retraining

■ ■ ■

Candidates' answers to Question 8

Candidate A

Attribution theory is where results are attributed to two types of factors:
- internal and stable factors that the player can control
- external unstable factors that are beyond the control of the performer

If the performer has low self-confidence because they lost many games in the previous season, the coach could help them in their long-term training by blaming these losses on external and unstable factors that they could not control.

This candidate defines attribution theory but does not really discuss how the coach could use this theory. The candidate has not, therefore, answered the question set. 1 mark is awarded for stating that the coach could attribute the losses to external factors.

Candidate B

A performer with low self-esteem will need to undergo attribution retraining during the long-term preparation phase. The coach would use this retraining to get the performer to concentrate on what are called the 'controllables' — these are internal factors, such as fitness levels and skill, which the player can work on in training and perfect so that when they compete they know they are prepared as best they can be.

The coach needs to get the player to feel that good performances and victories are the result of internal factors. They will tell the player that they won because they

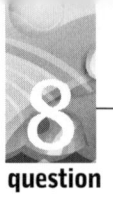

were good enough and had prepared well. Equally they can warn them that if they don't train hard enough then they will underperform.

Losses should be attributed to unstable and external factors that the player and coach cannot control — these would include factors such as the weather or the performance of the other team.

🖉 This answer scores the maximum 4 marks. The candidate clearly states the methods a coach would use in developing the confidence of the player. Good use of practical examples helps to back up the points.

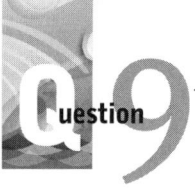

Question 9

Elite sports systems

Explain, using examples, the two models of elite sport found around the world.

(6 marks)

■ ■ ■

The marking points are given below. A maximum of 3 marks is available for an explanation of the centralised model, and 3 marks for the decentralised model (including 1 mark for each model correctly identified). However, note that examples *must* be given in order to gain marks.

The centralised model:

- Elite sports are supported via the state
- A central body oversees the management of the country's elite sports programme
- Public sector funding provides sports science support, elite training facilities
- Athletes' personal funding comes from the public sector
- Examples include the Australian/French/Chinese/former East German elite sports systems

The decentralised model:

- No single agency takes control of elite sports system
- Elite sport is supported through higher education institutions
- Funding for facilities and support comes from a variety of sources such as the private sector and voluntary sector funding from lotteries, etc.
- Athletes' personal funding comes from the private sector such a sponsorship or lottery funding
- Examples include the American and British elite sports systems

■ ■ ■

Candidates' answers to Question 9

Candidate A

There are two basic elite sports systems found in the world.

Centralised elite sports system

- The state takes control of elite sport.
- Most of the funding comes from the state or the public sector.
- Athletes are supported through a national system of sports institutes where they can train and receive sports science support.
- Examples include the old East German elite sports system and the current system in China.

Decentralised elite sports system

- The state has no central control of elite sport.
- Most of the funding comes from the private or voluntary sectors.

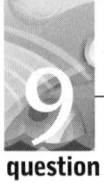

- Athletes train and receive sport science support through universities and colleges.
- The best example of a decentralised elite sports system is the USA.

⌦ This answer scores the maximum 6 marks. The candidate has clearly identified both systems, made relevant points and given global examples of each system. This bulleted style of answer can be an effective way of answering these shorter mark questions — but you need to make sure that each statement makes sense.

Candidate B

The centralised model is where elite sports are supported via the state, which appoints a central body to oversee the management of the country's elite sports programme. In this type of system, the majority of funding for sports science support, elite training facilities and also athletes' personal funding comes from the public sector.

The decentralised model is where no single agency takes control, but there is an elite sports system that is often based around higher education institutions. Here the funding for elite sport comes from the private sector through things such as sponsorship and advertising.

⌦ Though this answer includes some relevant points it does not contain any examples. The candidate has therefore failed to answer the question set and, unfortunately, does not receive any marks. This highlights again why it is so important to read the question carefully, several times, to make sure you know what you have to do.

Question 10

Use of holding camps

Discuss the scientific principles behind the use of holding camps prior to global sports competitions. (12 marks)

■ ■ ■

The mark scheme is shown in the table below.

Level	Mark	Descriptor
	0	No rewardable material
Level 1	1–3	Candidates will produce brief and narrative answers, making simple statements, showing little relevance to the question. The material will be mostly generalised with no attempt at the analytical demands of the question. The skills needed to produce effective writing will not normally be present. The writing may have some coherence and will be generally comprehensible, but will lack both clarity and organisation. There will be a high incidence of syntactical and/or spelling errors.
Level 2	4–6	Candidates will produce statements with some development in the form of mostly accurate and relevant factual material. There will be some attempt at analysis, with limited success. The range of skills needed to produce effective writing is likely to be limited. There are likely to be passages which lack clarity and proper organisation. Frequent syntactical and/or spelling errors are likely to be present.
Level 3	7–9	Candidates' answers will show some understanding of the focus of the question and will be broadly analytical. They will, however, include material which is descriptive, and thus only implicitly relevant to the question's focus, or which strays from that focus. The candidate will demonstrate most of the skills needed to produce effective extended writing but there will be lapses in organisation. Some syntactical and/or spelling errors are likely to be present.
Level 4	10–12	Candidates will offer an analytic response which is sustained and relates well to the focus of the question, and addresses the key issues contained in it. The analysis will be supported by accurate factual material, which is relevant to the question. The skills needed to produce convincing extended writing are in place, with good/excellent organisation and clarity. Very few syntactical and/or spelling errors may be found.

■ ■ ■

Candidates' answers to Question 10

Candidate A

Holding camps work towards the idea of sports preparation both on a physiological and psychological degree. They are used for teams to get together as a group

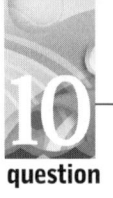

as well as individually to get to an optimum level of performance before a global sports competition such as a World Cup begins.

Skill-based exercises could be used to build up the essential skills needed for specific areas of the game as well as building up fitness levels.

The performers will also have time to be videoed and analysed so that they can increase the quality of performance. At the holding camp they will have access to top advice and help including equipment, sports medicine and psychologists.

In terms of psychology the holding camps allow the individuals in the teams to get mentally prepared for competition. Motivation talks from the coaches and team psychologists can help increase the self-efficacy of the players.

At the holding camp the coaches can also help the players deal with stress and anxiety by using techniques and strategies to overcome the anxiety of preparing for a global sports competition and deal with the rise in arousal. These techniques may include the use of relaxation strategies, using music or breathing techniques, which help the players stay calm and reach the right level of arousal.

By preparing players and combining them as a team they can all socially interact and understand the importance of working as a team.

Another thing that can be controlled during the time at the holding camp is the diet of the performers. Depending on the sports the athletes can build up muscle through protein-rich diets. They can build up their glycogen stores through carbo-loading and just generally being more aware of how much they are eating.

Being together as a team creates pride and the feeling that they want to play well — so in terms of motivation holding camps have a positive impact. The idea of holding camps is not only to build up team morale but to help the players prepare physically, psychologically and technically.

e This candidate does make an attempt at answering the question and makes reference to holding camps throughout their answer — though there are no specific examples given. The main problem is that many of the points relate to long-term preparation and adaptation, such as diet and fitness, which would not occur in a holding camp. Valid points are made relating to developing team bonding but these are repeated several times. The general structure of the answer is good but needs more detail and discussion. This answer would score in band 2 of the mark scheme.

Candidate B

Holding camps are useful in allowing performers to acclimatise to the environment in which their global sports competition is being held. They are used in the short-term preparation phase allowing teams and squads to get together and 'tweak' and focus on their final preparation and training.

The change of environment can include temperature and also time differences, which can create jet lag. This is a major reason why teams travel to a holding camp before competing in a country on the other side of the world. For example, the GB Olympic team had a holding camp in Macau — an island near China — in the final phase of preparation before the Beijing Olympics in 2008. The team went there 3 weeks before the Olympics so they could get over the jet lag and get used to the conditions.

Another reason is that they use the 3 weeks before competition, such as the football World Cup, to get the team eating the right type of diet to ensure that their energy stores are as full as possible. This will normally include carbo-loading — eating a diet with over 70% of carbohydrate. The England football team would also be using creatine supplements in this final phase at the holding camps to ensure that their ATP-PC stores are fully stocked. When teams are playing in humid areas, such as at the 2002 FIFA World Cup in Japan, hydration is also very important and a 1% drop in a player's fluid level can lead to a 10% drop in performance. The time at the holding camp can be used to get the level of fluid intake right and allow the players to adjust to the conditions — during training and practice games, players will be weighed and the physiologists will be able to work out how much fluid each player is losing and therefore how much fluid they need to take in.

Players will also benefit psychologically from the time spent at the holding camp. It will give them the opportunity to visit the venues and get to know what they are like — they can then use imagery techniques to help them prepare for their competition, running through their start and tactics.

Often, teams will be able to train in the venue so that they get a feel for the ground and the pitch. This may be important for goal kickers at the rugby World Cup to get used to the conditions in the stadium and work out any wind flow which may affect their kicking — for rugby and football teams the actual grass type and condition may determine what type of boots or studs they will wear during their games.

Time at the holding camp will also generate team bonding — getting used to each other and developing a good team spirit as well as shared set of goals for the tournament. This is particularly good for teams such as the Australian cricket team when they prepare for the next Ashes series in 2009 as they need to learn to work well as a team.

🖉 This candidate shows a good understanding of the use of holding camps. A range of points is made and many are backed up with direct reference to specific examples of global sports competitions, which is a really good idea. The candidate also covers physiological, psychological and technical points, which is what the longer mark questions will require you to do in your examination.

The general structure of the answer is good, though it does seem to end a little abruptly — it would be nice to see a summary at the end that brings together the key points. It is good practice to read the question again before starting your summary and then make specific reference to it in your final points in order to ensure that you are answering the question set.

This candidate would score at the bottom of band 4 of the mark scheme.

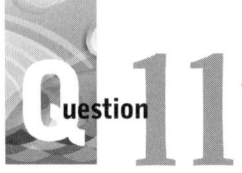

Question 11

Technology in sport

'Technology is now a necessary part of elite sports preparation.'

Discuss the positive and negative impact of technology in global sport. (12 marks)

■ ■ ■

The mark scheme is shown on p. 75.

■ ■ ■

Candidates' answers to Question 11

Candidate A

Technology and its use in sport is a key contemporary issue as people are constantly developing new things and making new advances that will result in new world records and improved performances. However, whether this is a good thing remains a constant debate — is it natural ability or the new technology that is making the athletes produce better performances year on year?

Technology in sport has had many positive effects, for example photo finishes and more accurate timing methods mean that we have the ability to record and analyse performances much more efficiently. It has also meant that new equipment can be produced, for examples hurdles that fall over when hit so as not to hurt the athletes. Clothing is also an element of technology where it could be described as having a negative element, for example if it is the shoe that is making the athlete so fast rather than the athlete themselves.

Scientific research is linked to developments in technology — for example, how areas of higher altitude can provide people with physiological adaptations. In the past athletes would have to travel to areas of high altitude to train there — Paula Radcliffe would go and do altitude training in her close season — whereas now hypoxic chambers are used by athletes to recreate the effects of altitude. This is called live low and train high. But this may be an unfair advantage as only athletes from richer countries will be able to afford to use this expensive type of technology.

Drugs and their technological development have also had a negative impact on global sport. Many athletes such as Dwain Chambers and Marion Jones have tested positive for using illegal drugs — it is interesting that in the case of Marion Jones she was embracing new technology as she wore the new Nike 'swift suit' and won many races and broke many world records. However, it was later found out that she had been using drugs and therefore her records and medals have been withdrawn. This shows different parts of the technological influences and how at first it showed a positive impact but then was overriden with the negative impact of technology in sport.

I think the main argument that makes people suggest that technology is having a negative impact on sport is that technology may make someone better that they actually are. This does not give an equal playing field for athletes. However if everyone or the vast majority of athletes are doing it then it can be argued that it does not matter.

ℓ This candidate successfully discusses both sides of the issue and backs up the points made with some examples, though these could be further developed. An attempt at summing up the main points gives a conclusion to the response. The writing quality could be improved. However, overall the answer includes a number of original and valid points and would score in band 3 of the mark scheme.

Candidate B

Technology is having a more positive impact on sport than a negative one. Some sports are more reliant on technology than others, for example yachting and motor racing. Another key benefit of technology is the facilities that are used. Most modern sports arenas are fitted with air con and heating — some have retractable roofs. Artificial pitches for football and hockey benefit performers a lot.

Ergogenic aids are things that increase a player's performance to a higher level than normally expected. The range of ergogenic aids is immense: supplements and drugs, hypnosis, training-monitoring equipment. Drugs such as amphetamines and caffeine lead to an increase in energy levels and decrease the sense of fatigue and increase arousal.

Sport science is another technological benefit — this is the application of any type of science to sport. Examples of these are specialist facilities and sports equipment. Another example is pupils being identified at a young age and then trained in a specific sport.

With technology getting so good, athletes have become dependent on the use of feedback, especially for feedback of performance. Footballers are now dependent on Prozone — this records exactly what each player does during a game and allows coaches to look at tactics.

ℓ This candidate gives a more limited view of technology. The answer lacks balance as it focuses only on the possible benefits of the use of technology in sport. The points made are limited and are not backed up with specific examples. Overall, the answer is a little muddled and would score in band 2 of the mark scheme.